INTRODUCTION

It is said that one of the characteristics of a profession is that it has a unique vocabulary, and health information management is no exception. This *Pocket Glossary for Health Information Management and Technology* is a compilation of the concepts and terms commonly used by professionals in the health information management (HIM) field. The *Pocket Glossary* brings these all together in one convenient reference for use by HIM practitioners, educators, students, researchers, and any healthcare professional with an interest in HIM practice. Terms and concepts reflect the breadth of practice drawing from the fields of medicine, healthcare management, computer science, and their application to health information management and technology.

This versatile desk reference is used to:

1. Define and explain the terms and concepts of the field
2. Explain emerging issues in healthcare
3. Provide preferred terms and synonyms to frame research
4. Understand the subject headings that frame HIM practice
5. Explain commonly used acronyms and abbreviations

DEVELOPMENT OF THE *POCKET GLOSSARY*

This reference was developed through comprehensive review of the books and articles of the HIM field and publications from other relevant healthcare domains. Each term was added because of its importance to the field and its value as a subject heading in health information management, including health information technology and informatics fields of study. Terms are updated biannually to reflect the expansion and emerging issues related to the healthcare industry.

This revision of the *Pocket Glossary for Health Information Management and Technology* was reviewed thoroughly by practitioners and educators in the field to ensure that it includes accurate and current technical content. Every attempt was made to capture the scope of specialty practice areas in HIM. It was designed to be a useful and useable reference tool for everyone who works—or aspires to work—in this exciting field.

FORMAT OF THE *POCKET GLOSSARY*

For ease of use, the *Pocket Glossary* is organized with many assists:

1. The terms are arranged alphabetically
2. A "See" or "also called" instruction directs you to related term or terms
3. Acronyms are integrated into the alphabetic glossary and a "See" reference gets you to the correct spelled-out term with its definition
4. Concepts that are numbers are spelled out and found in alphabetic order

Pocket Glossary
for
Health Information Management
and Technology

Third Edition

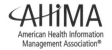

American Health Information
Management Association®

ISBN 978-1-58426-314-2
AHIMA Product No. AB105211

AHIMA Professional Practice Resource Staff
Ashley Sullivan, ASSISTANT EDITOR
Claire Blondeau, MBA, SENIOR EDITOR
Katie Greenock, MS, EDITORIAL AND PRODUCTION COORDINATOR
Ken Zielske, DIRECTOR OF PUBLICATIONS

American Health Information Management Association
233 North Michigan Avenue, 21st Floor
Chicago, Illinois 60601-5809
www.ahima.org

AHIMA took great care to capture all or most of the relevant terms in healthcare today; however, we recognize that the healthcare industry is changing at a rapid rate and we may have missed definitions. This publication is not a static resource; it will grow and change and these changes will be reflected in future editions.

Please help us make this *the* essential reference for the field by sharing your comments and suggestions. These may be suggestions for additional terms or concepts, or suggested revisions to any of the terms and concepts and their definitions. Please direct these to:

AHIMA Press Editor
American Health Information Management Association
233 North Michigan Avenue, 21st floor
Chicago, IL 60601-5800

Or by e-mail to publications@ahima.org

Acknowledgements

This *Pocket Glossary* is the collaborative effort of many. We thank the many authors who directly or indirectly contributed to this *Pocket Glossary*. We thank the reviewers who guided our team throughout its writing. We thank those involved in workgroups, volunteers, authors, and the AHIMA professional practice staff. Together they have made an important contribution to the body of knowledge for the profession.

GLOSSARY

AAAASF: *See* **American Association for Accreditation of Ambulatory Surgery Facilities**

AAAHC: *See* **Accreditation Association for Ambulatory Health Care**

AAHP: *See* **American Association of Health Plans**

AAMC: *See* **Association of American Medical Colleges**

AAMRL: *See* **American Association of Medical Record Librarians**

AAPC: *See* **American Academy of Professional Coders**

AAPPO: *See* **American Association of Preferred Provider Organizations**

Abbreviated Injury Scale (AIS): A set of numbers used in a trauma registry to indicate the nature and severity of injuries by body system

Abbreviations: Shortened forms of words or phrases; in healthcare, when there is more than one meaning for an approved abbreviation, only one meaning should be used or the context in which the abbreviation is to be used should be identified

ABC: *See* **activity-based costing**

ABC Codes: A terminology created by Alternative Link that describes alternative medicine, nursing, and other integrative healthcare interventions

Aberrancy: Services in medicine that deviate from what is typical in comparison to the national norm

Ability (achievement) tests: Tests used to assess the skills an individual already possesses; *Also called* **performance tests**

ABN: *See* **advance beneficiary notice**

Abnormal Involuntary Movement Scale (AIMS): A standardized form that can be used in facilities to document involuntary movements

Abortion: The expulsion or extraction of all (complete) or any part (incomplete) of the placenta or membranes, without an identifiable fetus or with a live-born infant or a stillborn infant weighing less than 500 grams

Absolute frequency: The number of times that a score of value occurs in a data set

Abstract: Brief summary of the major parts of a research study

Abstracting: 1. The process of extracting information from a document to create a brief summary of a patient's illness, treatment, and outcome 2. The process of extracting elements of data from a source document or database and entering them into an automated system

Abuse: Provider, supplier, and practitioner practices that are inconsistent with accepted sound fiscal, business, or medical practices that directly or indirectly may result in unnecessary costs to the program, improper payment, services that fail to meet professionally recognized standards of care or are medically unnecessary, or services that directly or indirectly result in adverse patient outcomes or delays in appropriate diagnosis or treatment

Abuses: Coding errors that occur without intent to defraud the government

Accept assignment: A term used to refer to a provider's or a supplier's acceptance of the allowed charges (from a fee schedule) as payment in full for services or materials provided

Acceptance testing: Final review during EHR implementation to ensure that all tests have been performed and all issues have been resolved; usually triggers the final payment for the system and when a maintenance contract becomes effective

Acceptance theory of authority: A management theory based on the principle that employees have the freedom to choose whether they will follow managerial directions

Access: 1. The ability of a subject to view, change, or communicate with an object in a computer system 2. One of the rights protected by the Privacy Rule; an individual has a right of access to inspect and obtain a copy of his or her own PHI that is contained in a designated record set, such as a health record

Access control: 1. A computer software program designed to prevent unauthorized use of an information resource 2. The process of designing, implementing, and monitoring a system for guaranteeing that only individuals who have a legitimate need are allowed to view or amend specific data sets

Access control grid: A tabular representation of the levels of authorization granted to users of a computer system's information and resources

Access control system: A system that defines who has access to what information in a computer system and specifies each user's rights and/or restrictions with respect to that information

Accession number: A number assigned to each case as it is entered in a cancer registry

Accession registry: A list of cases in a cancer registry in the order in which they were entered

Accidents/incidents: Those mishaps, misfortunes, mistakes, events, or occurrences that can happen during the normal daily routines and activities in the long-term care setting

Accommodating: In business, the practice whereby one party in a conflict or disagreement gives in to the other party as a temporary solution

Account: A subdivision of assets, liabilities, and equities in an organization's financial management system

Accountability: 1. The state of being liable for a specific activity 2. All information is attributable to its source (person or device)

Accountable: Required to answer to a supervisor for performance results

Accountable Care Organization (ACO): An organization of healthcare providers accountable for the quality, cost, and overall care of Medicare beneficiaries who are assigned and enrolled in the traditional fee-for-service program

Accountable health plan: *See* **integrated provider organization**

Accounting: 1. The process of collecting, recording, and reporting an organization's financial data 2. A list of all disclosures made of a patient's health information

Accounting entity: The business structure, including the activities and records to be maintained for the preparation of an individual organization's financial statements

Accounting of disclosures: HIPAA requirement to list, upon patient request, all disclosures that meet the criteria. Currently, this does not require accounting for disclosures for treatment, payment, and healthcare operations (TPO), but under ARRA this changes to include these disclosures; awaiting final regulations

Accounting period: The entire process of identifying and recording a transaction and ultimately reporting it as part of an organization's financial statement

Accounting rate of return: The projected annual cash inflows, minus any applicable depreciation, divided by the initial investment

Accounts Not Selected for Billing Report: A daily financial report used to track the many reasons why accounts may not be ready for billing

Accounts payable (A/P): Records of the payments owed by an organization to other entities

Accounts receivable (A/R): 1. Records of the payments owed to the organization by outside entities such as third-party payers and patients 2. Department in a healthcare facility that manages the accounts owed to the facility by customers who have received services but whose payment is made at a later date

Accreditation: 1. A voluntary process of institutional or organizational review in which a quasi-independent body created for this purpose periodically evaluates the quality of the entity's work against preestablished written criteria 2. A determination by an accrediting body that an eligible organization, network, program, group, or individual complies with applicable standards 3. The act of granting approval to a healthcare organization based on whether the organization has met a set of voluntary standards developed by an accreditation agency

Accreditation Association for Ambulatory Health Care (AAAHC): A professional organization that offers accreditation programs for ambulatory and outpatient organizations such as single-specialty and multispecialty group practices, ambulatory surgery centers, college/university health services, and community health centers

Accreditation Commission for Health Care (ACHC): An organization that provides quality standards and accreditation programs for home health and other healthcare organizations

Accreditation organization: A professional organization that establishes the standards against which healthcare organizations are measured and conducts periodic assessments of the performance of individual healthcare organizations

Accreditation standards: Preestablished statements of the criteria against which the performance of participating healthcare organizations will be assessed during a voluntary accreditation

Accredited Standards Committee X12 (ASC X12): A committee of the American National Standards Institute (ANSI) responsible for the development and maintenance of electronic data interchange (EDI) standards for many industries. The ASC "X12N" is the subcommittee of ASC X12 responsible for the EDI health insurance administrative transactions such as 837 Institutional Health Care Claim and 835 Professional Health Care Claim forms

Accrediting body: A professional organization that establishes the standards against which healthcare organizations are measured and conducts periodic assessment of the performance of individual healthcare organizations

Accrete: The term used by Medicare regarding the process of adding new members to a health plan

Accrual accounting: A method of accounting that requires business organizations to report income in the period earned and to deduct expenses in the period incurred

Accrue: The process of recording known transactions in the appropriate time period before cash payments/receipts are expected or due

Accuracy: The extent to which information reflects the true, correct, and exact description of the care that was delivered with respect to both content and timing

ACDIS: *See* **Association of Clinical Documentation Improvement Specialists**

ACGs: *See* **adjusted clinical groups**

ACH: *See* **automated clearinghouse**

ACHE: *See* **American College of Healthcare Executives**

Acid-test ratio: A ratio in which the sum of cash plus short-term investments plus net current receivables is divided by total current liabilities

Acknowledgement: A form that provides a mechanism for the resident to recognize receipt of important information

ACOG: American College of Obstetrics and Gynecology

Acquired immunodeficiency syndrome (AIDS): A retroviral disease caused by infection with human immunodeficiency virus (HIV)

Acquisition: One healthcare entity purchase of another healthcare entity in order to acquire control of all of its assets

ACR-NEMA: *See* **American College of Radiology-National Electrical Manufacturers Association**

ACS: *See* **American College of Surgeons**

Actinotherapy: The use of ultraviolet light therapy in the treatment of skin diseases

Action plan: A set of initiatives that are to be undertaken to achieve a performance improvement goal

Action steps: Specific plans an organization intends to accomplish in the near future as an effort toward achieving its long-term strategic plan

Active listening: The application of effective verbal communication skills as evidenced by the listener's restatement of what the speaker said

Active membership: Individuals interested in the AHIMA purpose and willing to abide by the Code of Ethics are eligible for active membership. Active members in good standing shall be entitled to all membership privileges including the right to vote

Active record: A health record of an individual who is a currently hospitalized inpatient or an outpatient

Activities of daily living (ADL): The basic activities of self-care, including grooming, bathing, ambulating, toileting, and eating

Activity-based budget: A budget based on activities or projects rather than on functions or departments

Activity-based costing (ABC): An economic model that traces the costs or resources necessary for a product or customer

Activity date or status: The element in the chargemaster that indicates the most recent activity of an item

Actor: The role a user plays in a system

Actual charge: 1. A physician's actual fee for service at the time an insurance claim is submitted to an insurance company, a government payer, or a health maintenance

organization; may differ from the allowable charge
2. Amount provider actually bills a patient, which may
differ from the allowable charge

Acute care: Medical care of a limited duration that is provided in an inpatient hospital setting to diagnose and/
or treat an injury or a short-term illness

Acute care prospective payment system: The Medicare
reimbursement methodology system referred to as the
inpatient prospective payment system (IPPS). Hospital providers subject to the IPPS utilize the Medicare
Severity Diagnosis Related Groups (MS-DRGs) classification system, which determines payment rates

ADA: *See* **American Dental Association**

ADA: *See* **Americans with Disabilities Act**

ADFM: Active duty family member; a designation used
under TRICARE

Ad hoc committee: A group of individuals who join together
to solve a particular task or problem

Addendum: A late entry added to a health record to provide
additional information in conjunction with a previous entry. The late entry should be timely and bear the
current date and reason for the additional information
being added to the health record

Addition of entries: Changes to the health record in the
form of late entries, amendments, or addenda

Add-on codes: In CPT coding, add-on codes are referred
to as additional or supplemental procedures. Add-on
codes are indicated with a "+" symbol and are to be
reported in addition to the primary procedure code.
Add-on codes are not to be reported as stand-alone
codes and are exempt from use of the –51 modifier

Addressable standards: The implementation specifications of the HIPAA Security Rule that are designated
"addressable" rather than "required"; to be in compliance with the rule, the covered entity must implement
the specification as written, implement an alternative,
or document that the risk for which the addressable
implementation specification was provided either does
not exist in the organization, or exists with a negligible
probability of occurrence

Adjunct diagnostic or therapeutic unit: An organized unit
of an inpatient hospital (other than an operating room,
delivery room, or medical care unit) with facilities
and personnel to aid physicians in the diagnosis and

treatment of illnesses or injuries through the performance of diagnostic or therapeutic procedures; *Also called* **ancillary unit**

Adjusted clinical groups (ACGs): A classification system that groups individuals according to resource requirements and reflects the clinical severity differences among the specific groups; formerly called ambulatory care groups

Adjusted historic payment base (AHPB): The weighted average prevailing charge for a physician service applied in a locality for 1991 and adjusted to reflect payments for services with charges below the prevailing charge levels and other payment limits; determined without regard to physician specialty and reviewed and updated yearly since 1992

Adjusted hospital autopsy rate: The proportion of hospital autopsies performed following the deaths of patients whose bodies are available for autopsy

Adjustment: The process of writing off an unpaid balance on a patient account to make the account balance

ADL: *See* **activities of daily living**

Administrative agencies: Executive branch agencies; source of administrative law

Administrative agency tribunals: A form of alternative dispute resolution in which tribunals are created by statute or the Constitution to hear disputes arising from administrative law

Administrative controls: Policies and procedures that address the management of computer resources

Administrative data: Coded information contained in secondary records, such as billing records, describing patient identification, diagnoses, procedures, and insurance

Administrative information: Information used for administrative and healthcare operations purposes, such as billing and quality oversight

Administrative information systems: A category of healthcare information systems that supports human resources management, financial management, executive decision support, and other business-related functions

Administrative law: A body of rules and regulations developed by various administrative entities empowered by Congress; falls under the umbrella of public law

Administrative law judge: A hearings officer who conducts appeal conflicts between providers of services, or beneficiaries, and Medicare contractors

Administrative management theory: A subdivision of classical management theory that emphasizes the total organization rather than the individual worker and delineates the major management functions

Administrative provisions: Documented, formal practices to manage data security measures throughout the healthcare organization

Administrative safeguards: Administrative actions such as policies and procedures and documentation retention to manage the selection, development, implementation, and maintenance of security measures to protect electronic protected health information and manage the conduct of the covered entity's or business associate's workforce in relation to the protection of that information

Administrative services: Business-related services provided by an insurance organization to self-insured employers or other parties according to an administrative services only contract (for example, actuarial support, benefit plan design, claims processing, data recovery and analysis, employee benefits communication, financial advice, medical care conversions, stop-loss coverage, and other services as requested)

Administrative services only (ASO) contract: An agreement between an employer and an insurance organization to administer the employer's self-insured health plan

Administrative simplification: A term referring to the Health Insurance Portability and Accountability Act (HIPAA) provisions which include standards for transactions and code sets that are used to exchange health data, standard identifiers for use on transactions, and privacy and security standards to protect personal health information. HIPAA included these administrative simplification provisions in order to improve the efficiency and effectiveness of the healthcare system.

Admissibility: The condition of being admitted into evidence in a court of law

Admission agreement: A legal contract signed by the resident that specifies the long-term care facility's responsibilities and fees for providing healthcare and other services

Admission date: The date the patient was admitted for inpatient care, outpatient service, or start of care. In the inpatient hospital setting, the admission date is the hospital's formal acceptance of a patient who is to receive healthcare services while receiving room, board, and continuous nursing services

Admissions and readmissions processing policy: A policy that provides the guidelines that are required when a resident is admitted or readmitted to the facility

Admission-discharge-transfer (ADT): The name given to software systems used in healthcare facilities that register and track patients from admission through discharge including transfers; usually interfaced with other systems used throughout a facility such as an electronic health record or lab information system

Admission type: The required classification used to indicate the priority of an admission/visit required for submitting claims using the electronic 837I format or the equivalent CMS-1450 claim form

Admission utilization review: A review of planned services (intensity of service) and/or a patient's condition (severity of illness) to determine whether care must be delivered in an acute care setting

Admitting diagnosis: A provisional description of the reason why a patient requires care in an inpatient hospital setting

Adoption: The decision to purchase, implement, and utilize an information system such as the EHR

ADR: *See* **adverse drug reaction**

ADS: *See* **alternative delivery system**

ADT: *See* **admission-discharge-transfer**

Adult day care: Group or individual therapeutic services provided during the daytime hours to persons outside their homes; usually provided for individuals with geriatric or psychiatric illnesses

Adult health questionnaire: *See* **patient history questionnaire**

Adult learning: Self-directed inquiry aided by the resources of an instructor, colleagues/fellow students, and educational materials

Advance beneficiary notice (ABN): A statement signed by the patient when he or she is notified by the provider, prior to a service or procedure being done, that Medicare may not reimburse the provider for the service, wherein the patient indicates that he will be responsible for any charges

Advanced decision support: Automated clinical practice guidelines that are built in to electronic health record systems and designed to support clinical decision making

Advance directive: A legal, written document that describes the patient's preferences regarding future healthcare or stipulates the person who is authorized to make medical decisions in the event the patient is incapable of communicating his or her preferences

Advanced practice registered nurse (APRN): The term being increasingly used by legislative and governing bodies to describe the collection of registered nurses that practice in the extended role beyond the normal role of basic registered nursing

Adverse action: A term used to refer to an action taken against a practitioner's clinical privileges or medical staff membership in a healthcare organization; *Also called* licensure disciplinary action

Adverse drug event: A patient injury resulting from a medication, either because of a pharmacological reaction to a normal dose, or because of a preventable adverse reaction to a drug resulting from an error

Adverse drug reaction (ADR): Unintended, undesirable, or unexpected effects of prescribed medications or of medication errors that require discontinuing a medication or modifying the dose, require initial or prolonged hospitalization, result in disability, require treatment with a prescription medication, result in cognitive deteriororation or impairment, are life threatening, result in death, or result in congenital anomalies

Adverse patient occurrences (APOs): Occurrences such as admission for adverse results of outpatient management, readmission for complications, incomplete management of problems on previous hospitalization, or unplanned removal, injury, or repair of an organ or structure during surgery; covered entities must have a system for concurrent or retrospective identification through medical chart–based review according to objective screening criteria

Adverse selection: A situation in which individuals who are sicker than the general population are attracted to a health insurance plan, with adverse effects on the plan's costs

Affiliated covered entity: Legally separate covered entities, affiliated by common ownership or control; for purposes of the Privacy Rule, these legally separate entities may refer to themselves as a single covered entity

Affinity diagram: A graphic tool used to organize and prioritize ideas after a brainstorming session

Affinity grouping: A technique for organizing similar ideas together in natural groupings

Aftercare: Healthcare services that are provided to a patient after a period of hospitalization or rehabilitation and are administered with the objective of improving or restoring health to the degree that aftercare is no longer needed

Against medical advice (AMA): The discharge status of patients who leave a hospital after signing a form that releases the hospital from any responsibility or who leave a hospital without notifying hospital personnel

Age Discrimination in Employment Act (1967): Federal legislation that prohibits employment discrimination against persons between the ages of 40 and 70 and restricts mandatory retirement requirements except where age is a bona fide occupational qualification

Agency for Healthcare Research and Quality (AHRQ): The branch of the US Public Health Service that supports general health research and distributes research findings and treatment guidelines with the goal of improving the quality, appropriateness, and effectiveness of healthcare services

Agenda for Change: An initiative undertaken by the Joint Commission that focused on changing the emphasis of the accreditation process from structure to outcomes

Aggregate data: Data extracted from individual health records and combined to form de-identified information about groups of patients that can be compared and analyzed

Aggregate information system: The combining of various data sets in order to compile overview or summary statistics

Aging of accounts: The practice of counting the days, generally in 30-day increments, from the time a bill was sent to the payer to the current day

AHA: *See* **American Hospital Association**

AHA Coding Clinic for HCPCS: The official coding advice resource for coding information on HCPCS CPT codes for hospital providers and certain HCPCS level II codes for hospitals, physicians, and other healthcare professionals

AHDI: *See* **Association for Healthcare Documentation Integrity**

AHIC: *See* **American Health Information Community**

AHIMA: *See* **American Health Information Management Association**

AHIMA Standards of Ethical Coding: The American Health Information Management Association's principles of professional conduct for coding professionals involved in diagnostic and/or procedural coding or other health record data abstraction

AHIP: *See* **America's Health Insurance Plans**

AHPB: *See* **adjusted historic payment base**

AHRQ: *See* **Agency for Healthcare Research and Quality**

AI: *See* **artificial intelligence**

AIS: *See* **abbreviated injury scale**

AIDS: *See* **acquired immunodeficiency syndrome**

AIMS: *See* **Abnormal Involuntary Movement Scale**

Alarm: A type of warning that is generated by an automated medical device

Alert: A software-generated warning that is based on a set of clinical rules built in to a healthcare information system

Algorithm: A procedure for solving a mathematical problem in a finite number of steps, which frequently involves repetition of an operation

Algorithmic translation: A process that involves the use of algorithms to translate or map clinical nomenclatures among each other or to map natural language to a clinical nomenclature or vice versa

Alias: A name added to, or substituted for, the proper name of a person; an assumed name

Alias policy: A policy that is implemented when resident confidentiality is require by the resident, family, or responsible party

ALJ: *See* **administrative law judge**

Allied health professional: A credentialed healthcare worker who is not a physician, nurse, psychologist, or pharmacist (for example, a physical therapist, dietitian, social worker, or occupational therapist)

Allowable charge: Average or maximum amount a third-party payer will reimburse providers for a service

All patient diagnosis-related groups (AP-DRGs): A case-mix system developed by 3M and used in a number of state reimbursement systems to classify non-Medicare discharges for reimbursement purposes

All patient refined diagnosis-related groups (APR-DRGs): An expansion of the inpatient classification system that includes four distinct subclasses (minor, moderate, major, and extreme) based on the severity of the patient's illness

ALOS: *See* **average length of stay**

Alphabetic filing system: A system of health record identification and storage that uses the patient's last name as the first component of identification and his or her first name and middle name or initial for further definition

Alphanumeric filing system: A system of health record identification and storage that uses a combination of alphabetic letters (usually the first two letters of the patient's last name) and numbers to identify individual records

Alteration: Modifying the natural anatomic structure of a body part without affecting the function of the body part. The principal purpose of this procedure is to improve the patient's appearance

Alternative delivery system (ADS): A type of healthcare delivery system in which health services are provided in settings such as skilled and intermediary facilities, hospice programs, nonacute outpatient programs, and home health programs, which are more cost-effective than in the inpatient setting

Alternative hypothesis: A hypothesis that states that there is an association between independent and dependent variables

Alternative Link: The original developer of the ABC codes

AMA: *See* **against medical advice**; **American Medical Association**

Ambulatory care: Preventive or corrective healthcare services provided on a nonresident basis in a provider's office, clinic setting, or hospital outpatient setting

Ambulatory care group (ACG): *See* **adjusted clinical groups**

Ambulatory care information system: A type of information system designed specifically for use and support in ambulatory care settings

Ambulatory care organization: A healthcare provider or facility that offers preventive, diagnostic, therapeutic, and rehabilitative services to individuals not classified as inpatients or residents

Ambulatory Care Quality Alliance: An organization consisting of a broad base of healthcare professionals who work collaboratively to improve healthcare quality and patient safety through performance measurement, data aggregation, and reporting in the ambulatory care setting

Ambulatory payment classification (APC): Hospital outpatient prospective payment system (OPPS). The classification is a resource-based reimbursement system. The payment unit is the ambulatory payment classification group (APC group)

Ambulatory payment classification group (APC group): Basic unit of the ambulatory payment classification (APC) system. Within a group, the diagnoses and procedures are similar in terms of resources used, complexity of illness, and conditions represented. A single payment is made for the outpatient services provided. APC groups are based on HCPCS/CPT codes. A single visit can result in multiple APC groups. APC groups consist of five types of service: significant procedures, surgical services, medical visits, ancillary services, and partial hospitalization. The APC group was formerly known as the ambulatory visit group (AVG) and ambulatory patient group (APG)

Ambulatory payment classification (APC) relative weight: A number reflecting the expected resource consumption of cases associated with each APC, relative to the average of all APCs, that is used in determining payment under the Medicare hospital outpatient prospective payment system (OPPS)

Ambulatory payment classification (APC) system: The Medicare reimbursement methodology system referred to as the hospital outpatient prospective payment system (OPPS). Hospital providers subject to the

OPPS utilize the ambulatory payment classification (APC) system, which determines payment rates

Ambulatory surgery center (ASC) payment rate: The Medicare ASC reimbursement methodology system referred to as the ambulatory surgery center (ASC) payment system. The ASC payment system is based on the ambulatory payment classifications (APCs) utilized under the hospital OPPS

Ambulatory surgery center or ambulatory surgical center (ASC): Under Medicare, an outpatient surgical facility that has its own national identifier; is a separate entity with respect to its licensure, accreditation, governance, professional supervision, administrative functions, clinical services, recordkeeping, and financial and accounting systems; has as its sole purpose the provision of services in connection with surgical procedures that do not require inpatient hospitalization; and meets the conditions and requirements set forth in the Medicare Conditions of Participation

Ambulatory surgical center (ASC) list: The Medicare ASC list which indicates procedures that are covered and paid if performed in the ASC setting

Ambulatory surgical center (ASC) services: ASC diagnostic and therapeutic procedures which can be safely performed outside a hospital setting

Amendment: Alteration of health information by modification, correction, addition, or deletion

Amendment request: The right of individuals to ask that a covered entity amend their health records, as provided in Section 164.526 of the Privacy Rule

American Academy of Professional Coders (AAPC): The American Academy of Professional Coders provides certified credentials to medical coders in physician offices, hospital outpatient facilities, ambulatory surgical centers, and in payer organizations

American Accreditation Healthcare Commission/ URAC: A healthcare quality improvement organization that offers managed care organizations, as well as other organizations, accreditation to validate quality healthcare, and provides education and measurement programs

American Association for Accreditation of Ambulatory Surgery Facilities (AAAASF): An organization that provides an accreditation program to ensure the quality and safety of medical and surgical care provided in ambulatory surgery facilities

American Association of Health Plans (AAHP): The trade organization for health maintenance organizations, preferred provider organizations, and other network-based health plans created by the merger of the Group Health Association of America and the American Managed Care and Review Association

American Association of Medical Record Librarians (AAMRL): The name adopted by the Association of Record Librarians of North America in 1944; precursor of the **American Health Information Management Association**

American Association of Preferred Provider Organizations (AAPPO): A national association composed of preferred provider organizations (PPOs) and affiliate organizations, which advocates for consumer awareness of their healthcare benefits and advocates for greater access, choice, and flexibility

American College of Healthcare Executives (ACHE): The national professional organization of healthcare administrators that provides certification services for its members and promotes excellence in the field

American College of Obstetricians and Gynecologists (ACOG): The professional association of medical doctors specializing in obstetrics and gynecology

American College of Radiology-National Electrical Manufacturers Association (ACR-NEMA): The professional organizations (ACR) and trade associations (NEMA) that work collaboratively to develop digital imaging standards

American College of Surgeons (ACS): The scientific and educational association of surgeons formed to improve the quality of surgical care by setting high standards for surgical education and practice

American College of Surgeons Commission on Cancer: The organization that approves cancer-related programs, including cancer registries and trauma centers

American Correctional Association (ACA): An organization that provides education, training, correctional certification, and accreditation for correctional healthcare organizations

American Dental Association (ADA): A professional dental association dedicated to the public's oral health, ethics, science, and professional advancement

American Health Information Community (AHIC): A public-private federal advisory committee associated with the Office of the National Coordinator that makes recommendations to the secretary on how to accelerate adoption of interoperable electronic health information technology

American Health Information Management Association (AHIMA): The professional membership organization for managers of health record services and healthcare information systems as well as coding services; provides accreditation, advocacy, certification, and educational services

American Hospital Association (AHA): The national trade organization that provides education, conducts research, and represents the hospital industry's interests in national legislative matters; membership includes individual healthcare organizations as well as individual healthcare professionals working in specialized areas of hospitals, such as risk management; one of the four Cooperating Parties on policy development for the use of ICD-9-CM

American Medical Association (AMA): The national professional membership organization for physicians that distributes scientific information to its members and the public, informs members of legislation related to health and medicine, and represents the medical profession's interests in national legislative matters; maintains and publishes the Current Procedural Terminology (CPT) coding system

American Medical Informatics Association (AMIA): A professional association for individuals, institutions, and corporations that promotes the development and use of medical informatics for patient care, teaching, research, and healthcare administration

American Medical Record Association (AMRA): The name adopted by the American Association of Medical Record Librarians in 1970; precursor of the **American Health Information Management Association**

American National Standards Institute (ANSI): An organization that governs standards in many aspects of public and private business; developer of the Health Information Technology Standards Panel

American Nurses Association (ANA): The national professional membership association of nurses that works for the improvement of health standards and the availability of healthcare services, fosters high professional standards for the nursing profession, and advances the economic and general welfare of nurses

American Occupational Therapy Association (AOTA): The nationally recognized professional association of more than 40,000 occupational therapists, occupational therapy assistants, and students of occupational therapy

American Osteopathic Association (AOA): The professional association of osteopathic physicians, surgeons, and graduates of approved colleges of osteopathic medicine that inspects and accredits osteopathic colleges and hospitals

American Physical Therapy Association (APTA): The national professional organization whose goal is to foster advancements in physical therapy practice, research, and education

American Psychiatric Association (APA): The international professional association of psychiatrists and related medical specialists that works to ensure humane care and effective treatment for all persons with mental disorders, including mental retardation and substance-related disorders

American Psychological Association (APA): The professional organization that aims to advance psychology as a science and profession and promotes health, education, and human welfare

American Recovery and Reinvestment Act of 2009 (ARRA): An economic stimulus package enacted by the 111th United States Congress in February 2009; signed into law by President Obama on February 17th, 2009; an unprecedented effort to jumpstart the economy, create/save millions of jobs, and put a down payment on addressing long-neglected challenges; an extraordinary response to a crisis unlike any since the Great Depression; includes measures to modernize our nation's infrastructure, enhance energy independence, expand educational opportunities, preserve and improve affordable health care, provide tax relief, and protect those in greatest need; *Also called* **Recovery Act; Stimulus**

American Society for Healthcare Risk Management (ASHRM): The professional society for healthcare risk management professionals that is affiliated with the American Hospital Association and provides educational tools and networking opportunities for its members

American Society for Quality (ASQ): A quality improvement organization whose members' interests are related to statistical process control, quality cost measurement and control, total quality management, failure analysis, and zero defects

American Society for Testing and Materials (ASTM): A national organization whose purpose is to establish standards on materials, products, systems, and services

American Society for Testing and Materials Committee E31 (ASTM E31)—Healthcare Informatics: A committee within the American Society for Testing and Materials that creates standards on the content, structure, and functionality of electronic health record systems, health information confidentiality policies and procedures, health data security, and the exchange of information across clinical systems, such as laboratory devices with information systems

American Society for Testing and Materials Standard E1384 (ASTM E1384)—Standard Guide for Description of Content and Structure of an Automated Primary Record of Care: A standard that identifies the basic information to be included in electronic health records and requires the information to be organized into categories

American Standard Code for Information Interchange (ASCII): Electronic code that represents text, which makes it possible to transfer data from one computer to another

Americans with Disabilities Act (ADA) of 1990: Federal legislation which ensures equal opportunity for and elimination of discrimination against persons with disabilities

America's Health Insurance Plans (AHIP): A national trade association representing companies providing health benefits to Americans; formerly known as the Health Insurance Association of America (HIAA)

AMIA: *See* **American Medical Informatics Association**

AMLOS: *See* **arithmetic mean length of stay**

AMRA: *See* **American Medical Record Association**

ANA: *See* **American Nurses Association**

Analog: Data or information that is *not* represented in an encoded, computer-readable format

Analysis: Review of health record for proper documentation and adherence to regulatory and accreditation standards

Analysis of discharged health records policy: A policy that outlines steps to be taken to process discharged resident records

Analysis phase: The first phase of the systems development life cycle during which the scope of the project is defined, project goals are identified, current systems are evaluated, and user needs are identified

Analysis session: The process of mining a data segment

Analyte: Any material or chemical substance subjected to analysis

Anatomical modifiers: Two-digit CPT codes that provide information about the exact body location of procedures, such as –LT, Left side, and –TA, Left great toe

Ancillary packaging: The inclusion of routinely performed support services in the reimbursement classification of a healthcare procedure or service

Ancillary services: 1. Tests and procedures ordered by a physician to provide information for use in patient diagnosis or treatment 2. Professional healthcare services such as radiology, laboratory, or physical therapy

Ancillary service visit: The appearance of an outpatient in a unit of a hospital or outpatient facility to receive services, tests, or procedures; ordinarily not counted as an encounter for healthcare services

Ancillary systems: Electronic systems that generate clinical information (such as laboratory information systems, radiology information systems, pharmacy information systems, and so on)

Ancillary unit: *See* **adjunct diagnostic or therapeutic unit**

Androgynous leadership: Leadership in which cultural stereotyped masculine and feminine styles are integrated into a more effective hybrid style

Anesthesia death rate: The ratio of deaths caused by anesthetic agents to the number of anesthesias administered during a specified period of time

Anesthesia report: The report that notes any preoperative medication and response to it, the anesthesia administered with dose and method of administration, the duration of administration, the patient's vital signs while under anesthesia, and any additional products given the patient during a procedure

Anesthetic risk: The risk of harm resulting from the administration of anesthetic agents

ANN: *See* **artificial neural network**

ANSI: *See* **American National Standards Institute**

Antegrade: Extending or moving forward

Antipsychotic Dyskinesia Identification System: One of several standardized forms for assessing and documenting abnormal movements (of face, eyes, mouth/tongue, or body) that may occur in the course of treatment with some psychotropic medications; *See also* **discus monitoring form**

Antipsychotic medications: Drugs that are used in the management of psychotic conditions, bipolar disorders, or major depression with psychotic features

Any and all records: A phrase frequently used by attorneys in the discovery phase of a legal proceeding. Subpoena-based requests containing this phrase may create a situation where the record custodian or provider's legal counsel can work to limit the records disclosed to those defined by a particular healthcare entity's legal health record. Typically, this is only during a subpoena phase, unless the information is legally privileged or similarly protected; the discovery phase of litigation probably can be used to request any and all relevant materials

AOA: *See* **American Osteopathic Association**

AOTA: *See* **American Occupational Therapy Association**

A/P: *See* **accounts payable**

APA: *See* **American Psychiatric Association**; **American Psychological Association**

APC: *See* **ambulatory payment classification**

APC group: *See* **ambulatory payment classification group**

APC grouper: Software programs that help coders determine the appropriate ambulatory payment classification for an outpatient encounter

APC relative weight: *See* **ambulatory payment classification relative weight**

APC system: *See* **ambulatory payment classification system**

AP-DRGs: *See* **all patient diagnosis-related groups**

API: *See* **application programming interface**

APOs: *See* **adverse patient occurrences**

Appeal: 1. A request for reconsideration of a denial of coverage or rejection of claim decision 2. The next stage in the litigation process after a court has rendered a verdict; must be based on alleged errors or disputes of law rather than errors of fact

Appellate court: Courts that hear appeals on final judgments of the state trial courts or federal trial courts

Append: The operation that results in adding information to documentation already in existence

Application controls: Security strategies, such as password management, included in application software and computer programs

Application programming interface (API): A set of definitions of the ways in which one piece of computer software communicates with another or a programmer makes requests of the operating system or another application; operates outside the realm of the direct user interface

Applications and data criticality analysis: A covered entity's formal assessment of the sensitivity, vulnerabilities, and security of its programs and the information it generates, receives, manipulates, stores, and/or transmits

Application service provider (ASP): A third-party service company that delivers, manages, and remotely hosts standardized applications software via a network through an outsourcing contract based on fixed, monthly usage, or transaction-based pricing

Applied artificial intelligence: An area of computer science that deals with algorithms and computer systems that exhibit the characteristics commonly associated with human intelligence

Applied healthcare informatics: Automated information systems applied to healthcare delivery business and workflow processes, including the diagnosis, therapy, and systems of managing health data and information within the healthcare setting

Applied research: A type of research that focuses on the use of scientific theories to improve actual practice, as in medical research applied to the treatment of patients

Appreciative inquiry: An organizational development technique in which successful practices are identified and expanded throughout the organization

APR: *See* **average payment rate**

APR-DRGs: *See* **all patient refined diagnosis-related groups**

APRN: *See* **advanced practice registered nurse**

APS: *See* **Attending Physician Statement**

APTA: *See* **American Physical Therapy Association**

Aptitude tests: Tests that assess an individual's general ability to learn a new skill

AQA Alliance: A broad-based coalition of physicians, consumers, purchasers, health insurance plans, and others who are committed to effectively and efficiently improve performance measurement, data aggregation, and reporting in the ambulatory care setting

A/R: *See* **accounts receivable**

AR: *See* **attributable risk**

Arbitration: A proceeding in which disputes are submitted to a third party or a panel of experts outside the judicial trial system

Architecture: The configuration, structure, and relationships of hardware (the machinery of the computer including input/output devices, storage devices, and so on) in an information system

Archival database: A historical copy of a database that is saved at a particular point in time. It is used to recover and/or restore the information in the database

Archive file: A file in a collection of files reserved for later research or verification for the purposes of security, legal processes, and/or backup

ARD: *See* **assessment reference date**

Arden syntax: A standard language for encoding medical knowledge representation for use in clinical decision support systems

Area of excellence: A describable skill, competence, or capability that a department or company cultivates to a level of proficiency

Arithmetic mean length of stay (AMLOS): The average length of stay for all patients

ARLNA: *See* **Association of Record Librarians of North America**

ARRA: *See* **American Recovery and Reinvestment Act of 2009 (ARRA)**

Artificial intelligence (AI): High-level information technologies used in developing machines that imitate human qualities such as learning and reasoning

Artificial neural network (ANN): A computational technique based on artificial intelligence and machine learning in which the structure and operation are inspired by the properties and operation of the human brain

ASA: American Society of Anesthesiologists

ASC: *See* **Accredited Standards Committee; ambulatory surgery center**

ASCII: *See* **American Standard Code for Information Interchange**

ASC list: *See* **ambulatory surgical center list**

ASC services: *See* **ambulatory surgical center services**

ASC X12: Accredited Standards Committee, Electronic Data Interchange; *See* **Accredited Standards Committee X12 (ASC X12)**

ASHRM: *See* **American Society for Healthcare Risk Management**

ASO contract: *See* **administrative services only contract**

ASP: *See* **application service provider**

ASQ: *See* **American Society for Quality**

Assembler: A computer program that translates assembly-language instructions into machine language

Assembly language: A second-generation computer programming language that uses simple phrases rather than the complex series of switches used in machine language

Assessment: The systematic collection and review of information pertaining to an individual who wants to receive healthcare services or enter a healthcare setting

Assessment completion date: According to the Centers for Medicare and Medicaid Services' instructions, the date by which a Minimum Data Set for Long-Term Care must be completed; that is, within 14 days of admission to a long-term care facility

Assessment final completion date: The date (within 32 days of the assessment's final completion date) on which the Centers for Medicare and Medicaid requires Minimum Data Set for Long-Term Care assessments to be electronically submitted to the facility's state Minimum Data Set for Long-Term Care database

Assessment indicator code: A component of the code used for Medicare billing by long-term care facilities

Assessment locking: A term that refers to the Centers for Medicare and Medicaid Services' requirement that long-term care facilities must encode Minimum Data Set assessments in a computerized file and edit the data items for compliance with data specifications

Assessment reference date (ARD): The date that sets the designated end point of resident observation for all staff participating in the assessment

Assets: The human, financial, and physical resources of an organization

Assignment: An agreement between a physician and CMS whereby a physician or supplier agrees to accept the Medicare-approved amount as payment in full for services or supplies provided under Part B. Medicare pays the physician or supplier 80 percent of the approved amount after the annual $100 deductible has been met; the beneficiary pays the remaining 20 percent

Assignment of benefits: The transfer of one's interest or policy benefits to another party; typically the payment of medical benefits directly to a provider of care

Assisted living: A type of freestanding long-term care facility where residents receive necessary medical services but retain a degree of independence

Association for Healthcare Documentation Integrity (AHDI): Formerly the American Association for Medical Transcription (AAMT), the AHDI has a model curriculum for formal educational programs that includes the study of medical terminology, anatomy and physiology, medical science, operative procedures, instruments, supplies, laboratory values, reference use and research techniques, and English grammar

Association of American Medical Colleges (AAMC): The organization established in 1876 to standardize the curriculum for medical schools in the United States and to promote the licensure of physicians

Association of Clinical Documentation Improvement Specialists (ACDIS): Formed in 2007 as a community in which clinical documentation improvement professionals could communicate resources and strategies to implement successful programs and achieve professional growth

Association of Record Librarians of North America (ARLNA): Organization formed 10 years after the beginning of the hospital standardization movement whose original objective was to elevate the standards of clinical recordkeeping in hospitals, dispensaries, and other healthcare facilities; precursor of the **American Health Information Management Association**

Association rule analysis (rule induction): The process of extracting useful if/then rules from data based on statistical significance; *See also* **rule induction**

Assumption coding: The practice of assigning codes on the basis of clinical signs, symptoms, test findings, or treatments without supporting physician documentation

Assumptions: Undetermined aspects of a project that are considered to be true (for example, assuming that project team members have the right skill set to perform their duties)

ASTM: *See* **American Society for Testing and Materials**

ASTM E1384: *See* **American Society for Testing and Materials Standard E1384—Standard Guide for Description of Content and Structure of an Automated Primary Record of Care**

ASTM E31: *See* **American Society for Testing and Materials Committee E31—Healthcare Informatics**

ASTM International: Formerly known as the American Society for Testing and Materials, a system of standards developed primarily for various EHR management processes

ASTM Standard E1384-02a: Standard that identifies the content and structure for EHRs, covering all types of healthcare services, including acute care hospitals, ambulatory care, skilled nursing facilities, home healthcare, and specialty environments

Asynchronous: Occurring at different times

Asynchronous transfer mode (ATM): A topology for transmitting data across large wide-area networks

Atlas System: A severity-of-illness system commonly used in the United States and Canada

ATM: *See* **asynchronous transfer mode**

At risk contract: A type of managed care contract between Medicare and a payer or a payer and a provider according to which patients receive care during the entire term of the contract even if actual costs exceed the payment established by the agreement

Attending physician: The physician primarily responsible for the care and treatment of a patient

Attending physician identification: The unique national identification number assigned to the clinician of record at discharge who is responsible for the inpatient discharge summary

Attending Physician Statement (APS): The standardized insurance claim form created in 1958 by the Health Insurance Association of America and the American Medical Association; *See also* **COMB-1 form**

Attestation: The act of applying an electronic signature to the content showing authorship and legal responsibility for a particular unit of information

Attorney-client privilege: An understanding that protects communication between client and attorney

Attorney in fact: Agent authorized by an individual to make certain decisions, such as healthcare determinations, according to a directive written by the individual

Attributable risk (AR): A measure of the impact of a disease on a population (for example, measuring additional risk of illness as a result of exposure to a risk factor)

Attributes: 1. Data elements within an entity that become the column or field names when the entity relationship diagram is implemented as a relational database 2. Properties or characteristics of concepts; used in SNOMED CT to characterize and define concepts

Attrition: *See* **mortality**

Audioconferencing: A learning technique in which participants in different locations can learn together via telephone lines while listening to a presenter and looking at handouts or books

Audit: 1. A function that allows retrospective reconstruction of events, including who executed the events in question, why, and what changes were made as a result 2. To conduct an independent review of electronic system records and activities in order to test the adequacy and effectiveness of data security and data integrity procedures and to ensure compliance with established policies and procedures; *See also* **external review**

Auditability: The ability to do a methodical examination and verification of all information activities such as entering and accessing

Audit controls: The mechanisms that record and examine activity in information systems

Audit log: A chronological record of electronic system(s) activities that enables the reconstruction, review, and

examination of the sequence of events surrounding
or leading to each event and/or transaction from its
beginning to end. Includes who performed what event
and when it occurred

Audit reduction tool: Used to review the audit trail and
compare it to facility-specific criteria and eliminate
routine entries such as the periodic backups

Audit trail: 1. A chronological set of computerized records
that provides evidence of information system activity
(log-ins and log-outs, file accesses) used to determine
security violations 2. A record that shows who has
accessed a computer system, when it was accessed, and
what operations were performed; *See also* **audit log**

Auditing: The performance of internal and/or external
reviews (audits) to identify variations from established
baselines (for example, review of outpatient coding as
compared with CMS outpatient coding guidelines)

Authenticate: Confirm by signing

Authenticated evidence: Evidence that appears to be relevant and has been shown to have a baseline authenticity or trustworthiness

Authentication: 1. The process of identifying the source of
health record entries by attaching a handwritten signature, the author's initials, or an electronic signature
2. Proof of authorship that ensures, as much as possible, that log-ins and messages from a user originate
from an authorized source

Authenticity: The genuineness of a record, that it is what it
purports to be; information is authentic if proven to be
immune from tampering and corruption

Author: Person(s) who is (are) responsible and accountable
for the health information creation, content, accuracy,
and completeness for each documented event or health
record entry

Authority: The right to make decisions and take actions
necessary to carry out assigned tasks

Authorization: 1. The granting of permission to disclose
confidential information; as defined in terms of the
HIPAA Privacy Rule, an individual's formal, written
permission to use or disclose his or her personally
identifiable health information for purposes other
than treatment, payment, or healthcare operations 2. A
patient's consent to the disclosure of protected health

information (PHI); the form by which a patient gives consent to release of information

Authorization management: The process of protecting the security and privacy of the confidential data in a database

Authorization to disclose information: An authorization that allows the healthcare facility to verbally disclose or send health information to other organizations; *See also* **authorization**

Authorship: The origination or creation of recorded information attributed to a specific individual or entity acting at a particular time

Autoauthentication: 1. A procedure that allows dictated reports to be considered automatically signed unless the health information management department is notified of needed revisions within a certain time limit 2. A process by which the failure of an author to review and affirmatively either approve or disapprove an entry within a specified time period results in authentication

Autocoding: The process of extracting and translating dictated and then transcribed free-text data (or dictated and then computer-generated discrete data) into ICD-9-CM and CPT evaluation and management codes for billing and coding purposes

Autodialing system: A method used to automatically call and remind patients of upcoming appointments

Automated clearinghouse (ACH): An electronic network for the processing of financial transactions

Automated code assignment: Uses data that have been entered into a computer to automatically assign codes; uses natural language processing (NLP) technology—algorithmic (rules-based) or statistical—to read the data contained in a CPR

Automated codebook encoder: A type of encoder that mimics the codebook

Automated forms processing technology: Technology that allows users to electronically enter data into online digital forms and electronically extract data from online digital forms for data collection or manipulation; *See also* **e-forms technology**

Automatic log-off: A security procedure that ends a computer session after a predetermined period of inactivity

Autonomy: A core ethical principle centered on the individual's right to self-determination that includes respect for the individual; in clinical applications, the patient's right to determine what does or does not happen to him or her in terms of healthcare

Autopsy: The postmortem examinations of the organs and tissues of a body to determine the cause of death or pathological conditions

Autopsy rate: The proportion or percentage of deaths in a healthcare organization that are followed by the performance of autopsy

Autopsy report: Written documentation of the findings from a postmortem pathological examination

Availability: The accessibility for continuous use of data

Available for hospital autopsy: A situation in which the required conditions have been met to allow an autopsy to be performed on a hospital patient who has died

Average: The value obtained by dividing the sum of a set of numbers by the number of values

Average daily census: The mean number of hospital inpatients present in the hospital each day for a given period of time

Average duration of hospitalization: *See* **average length of stay**

Average length of stay (ALOS): The mean length of stay for hospital inpatients discharged during a given period of time

Average payment rate (APR): The amount of money the Centers for Medicare and Medicaid could pay a health maintenance organization for services rendered to Medicare recipients under a risk contract

Average record delinquency rate: The monthly average number of discharges divided by the monthly average number of delinquent records

Average wholesale price (AWP): The price commonly used when negotiating pharmacy contracts

Avoiding: In business, a situation where two parties in conflict ignore that conflict

Awareness training: Training designed to help individuals understand and respond to information technology concerns

AWP: *See* **average wholesale price**

Backbone: A high-speed medium used as the main trunk in a computer network to transmit high volumes of traffic

Back-end speech recognition (BESR): Specific use of SRT in an environment where the recognition process occurs after the completion of dictation by sending voice files through a server

Backscanning: The process of scanning past medical records into the system so that there is an existing database of patient information, making the system valuable to the user from the first day of implementation

Backup: The process of maintaining a copy of all software and data for use in the case that the primary source becomes compromised

Backward compatibility: The capability of a software or hardware product to work with earlier versions of itself

Bad debt: The receivables of an organization that are uncollectible

Balance billing: A reimbursement method that allows providers to bill patients for charges in excess of the amount paid by the patients' health plan or other third-party payer (not allowed under Medicare or Medicaid)

Balanced Budget Act (BBA) of 1997: Public Law 105-33 enacted by Congress on August 5, 1997, that mandated a number of additions, deletions, and revisions to the original Medicare and Medicaid legislation; the legislation that added penalties for healthcare fraud and abuse to the Medicare and Medicaid programs and also affected the hospital outpatient prospective payment system (HOPPS) and programs of all-inclusive care for elderly (PACE)

Balanced Budget Refinement Act (BBRA) of 1999: The amended version of the Balanced Budget Act of 1997 that authorized implementation of a per-discharge prospective payment system for care provided to Medicare beneficiaries by inpatient rehabilitation facilities

Balanced scorecard (BSC) methodology: A strategic planning tool that identifies performance measures related to strategic goals

Balance sheet: A report that shows the total dollar amounts in accounts, expressed in accounting equation format, at a specific point in time

Baldridge Award: A congressional award that recognizes excellence in several areas of business

Bandwidth: The range of frequencies a device or communication medium is capable of carrying

Bar chart: A graphic technique used to display frequency distributions of nominal or ordinal data that fall into categories; *Also called* **bar graph**

Barcode-enabled devices: Devices used throughout healthcare facilities that are designed to use barcodes for increased accuracy; *See also* **barcoding technology**

Barcode medication administration record (BC-MAR): System that uses barcoding technology for positive patient identification and drug information

Barcoding technology: A method of encoding data that consists of parallel arrangements of dark elements, referred to as bars, and light elements, referred to as spaces, and interpreting the data for automatic identification and data collection purposes

Bar graph: *See* **bar chart**

Baseline: The original estimates for a project's schedule, work, and cost

Baseline adjustment for volume and intensity of service: An adjustment to the conversion factor needed to fulfill the statutory budget neutrality requirement

Base (payment) rate: Rate per discharge for operating and capital-related components for an acute care hospital

Base year: Cost reporting period upon which a rate is based

Basic research: A type of research that focuses on the development and refinement of theories

Batch processing: The grouping of computer tasks to be run at one time; common in mainframe systems where the user did not interact with the computer in real time but, instead, data were often processed at night and produced time-delayed output

BBA of 1997: *See* **Balanced Budget Act of 1997**

BBRA of 1999: *See* **Balanced Budget Refinement Act of 1999**

BC/BS: *See* **Blue Cross and Blue Shield**

BCBSA: *See* **Blue Cross and Blue Shield Association**

BC/BS Service Benefit Plan: *See* **Blue Cross and Blue Shield Federal Employee Program (FEP)**

Beacon Community Cooperative Agreement Program: Provides funding to selected communities to build and strengthen their health information technology infrastructure and exchange capabilities. The program supports these communities at the cutting edge of EHR adoption and health information exchange to push them to a new level of sustainable healthcare quality and efficiency

Bed capacity: The number of beds that a facility has been designed and constructed to house

Bed complement: *See* **bed count**

Bed count: The number of inpatient beds set up and staffed for use on a given day; *Also called* **bed complement**

Bed count day: A unit of measure that denotes the presence of one inpatient bed (either occupied or vacant) set up and staffed for use in one 24-hour period

Bed occupancy ratio: The proportion of beds occupied, defined as the ratio of inpatient service days to bed count days during a specified period of time

Bed size: The total number of inpatient beds for which a facility is equipped and staffed to provide patient care services

Bed turnover rate: The average number of times a bed changes occupants during a given period of time

Behavioral description interview: An interview format that requires applicants to give specific examples of how they have performed a specific procedure or handled a specific problem in the past

Behavioral healthcare: A broad array of psychiatric services provided in acute, long-term, and ambulatory care settings; includes treatment of mental disorders, chemical dependency, mental retardation, and developmental disabilities, as well as cognitive rehabilitation services

Behavioral healthcare information: Information related to treatment for conditions such as mental disorders, mental retardation, and other developmental disabilities

Behavioral healthcare organization: An organization that can provide a wide array of services, including diagnosis and treatment for mental disorders, chemical dependency, mental retardation, developmental disabilities, and cognitive rehabilitative services in an acute, long-term, or ambulatory care setting

Belmont Report: A statement of ethical principles to prevent the unethical use of human subjects in research, sponsored by the Department of Health and Human Services

Bench trial: A trial in which a judge reviews the evidence and makes a determination, without a sitting jury

Benchmarking: The systematic comparison of the products, services, and outcomes of one organization with those of a similar organization; or the systematic comparison of one organization's outcomes with regional or national standards

Benchmarking survey: A survey in which a healthcare facility compares elements of its operation with those of similar healthcare facilities

Beneficence: A legal term that means promoting good for others or providing services that benefit others, such as releasing health information that will help a patient receive care or will ensure payment for services received

Beneficiary: An individual who is eligible for benefits from a health plan

Beneficiary-elected transfer: The elective transfer of a patient from one home health agency to another during a 60-day episode

Benefit: Healthcare service for which the healthcare insurance company will pay; *See* **covered expenses**

Benefit cap: Total dollar amount that a healthcare insurance company will pay for covered healthcare services during a specified period, such as a year or lifetime

Benefit level: The degree to which a person is entitled to receive services based on his or her contract with a health plan or an insurer

BESR: *See* **back-end speech recognition**

Best of breed: A vendor strategy used when purchasing an EHR that refers to system applications that are considered the best in their class

Best of fit: A vendor strategy used when purchasing an EHR in which all the systems required by the healthcare facility are available from one vendor

Best practice: Term used to refer to services that have been deemed effective and efficient with certain groups of clients

BI: *See* **business intelligence**

Bill drop: The point at which a bill is completed and electronically or manually sent to the payer

Bill hold period: The span of time during which a bill is suspended in the billing system awaiting late charges, diagnosis and/or procedure codes, insurance verification, or other required information

Billing audit: *See* **quantitative audit**

Bills of Mortality: Documents used in London during the 17th century to identify the most common causes of death

Bioethics: A field of study that applies ethical principles to decisions that affect the lives of humans, such as whether to approve or deny access to health information

Bioethics and privacy commissions: Commissions that US government has formed to specifically address issues related to privacy, electronic systems, and research; for example, in 1972–1973, the Health Education and Welfare (HEW) secretary established the Advisory Committee on Automated Personal Data Systems, the first attempt to establish fair information practices for automated personal data systems

Biofeedback: The process of providing visual or auditory evidence to a person on the status of an autonomic body function (such as the sounding of a tone when blood pressure is at a desirable level) so that he or she learns to exert control over the function

Biomedical research: The process of systematically investigating subjects related to the functioning of the human body

Biometric identification system: An identification system that analyzes biological data about users, such as voiceprints, fingerprints, handprints, retinal scans, faceprints, and full-body scans

Biometrics: The physical characteristics of users (such as fingerprints, voiceprints, retinal scans, iris traits) that systems store and use to authenticate identity before allowing the user access to a system

Biotechnology: The field devoted to applying the techniques of biochemistry, cellular biology, biophysics, and molecular biology to addressing practical issues related to human beings, agriculture, and the environment

BI-RADS: *See* **Breast Imaging Reporting and Data System Atlas**

Birth certificate: Paperwork that must be filed for every live birth regardless of where it occurred

Birth certificate information system: This software reports births occurring in the healthcare facility to the state health agency. The birth certificate information system software may be developed by the state or by a vendor

Birthday rule: A method of determining which insurance company is the primary carrier for dependents when both parents carry insurance on them. The rule states that the policyholder with the birthday earliest in the calendar year carries the primary policy for the dependents. If the policyholders are both born on the same day, the policy that has been in force the longest is the primary policy. Birth year has no relevance in this method

Birth weight: The weight of a neonate (expressed to the nearest gram) determined immediately after delivery or as soon thereafter as feasible

Birth weight of newborn (inpatient): The specific birth weight of the newborn, recorded in grams

Bit: The level of voltage (low or high) in a computer that provides the binary states of 0 and 1 that computers use to represent characters

Bitmapped data: Data made up of pixels displayed on a horizontal and vertical grid or matrix

Bivariate: An adjective meaning the involvement of two variables

Blanket authorization: An authorization for the release of confidential information from a certain point in time and any time thereafter

Blended learning: A training strategy that uses a combination of techniques—such as lecture, web-based training, or programmed text—to appeal to a variety of learning styles and maximize the advantages of each training method

Blended rate: A rate assigned to hospitals by the CMS based on cost of living, location, and services provided

Blitz team: A type of PI team that constructs relatively simple and quick "fixes" to improve work processes without going through the complete PI cycle

Block grant: Fixed amount of money given or allocated for a specific purpose, such as a transfer of governmental funds to cover health services

Blogs: Web logs that provide a web page where users can post text, images, and links to other websites

Blood and blood component usage review: Evaluation of how blood and blood components are used using the Joint Commission guidelines

Bloodborne pathogen: Infectious diseases such as HIV, hepatitis B, and hepatitis C that are transported through contact with infected body fluids such as blood, semen, and vomitus

Blue Cross and Blue Shield (BC/BS): The first prepaid healthcare plans in the United States; Blue Shield plans traditionally cover hospital care and Blue Cross plans cover physicians' services

Blue Cross and Blue Shield Association (BCBSA): The national association of state and local Blue Cross and Blue Shield plans

Blue Cross and Blue Shield Federal Employee Program (FEP): A federal program that offers a fee-for-service plan with preferred provider organizations and a point-of-service product; *Also called* **BC/BS Service Benefit Plan**

Board certified: A designation given to a physician or other health professional who has passed an exam from a medical specialty board and is thereby certified to provide care within that specialty

Boarder: An individual such as a parent, caregiver, or other family member who receives lodging at a healthcare facility but is not a patient

Boarder baby: A newborn who remains in the nursery following discharge because the mother is still hospitalized or a premature infant who no longer needs intensive care but remains for observation

Board of directors: The elected or appointed group of officials who bear ultimate responsibility for the successful operation of a healthcare organization; *Also called* board of governors; board of trustees

Body of Knowledge (BoK): The collected resources, knowledge, and expertise within and related to a profession

BoK: *See* **Body of Knowledge**

Boot-record infectors: *See* **system infectors**

Bounded rationality: The recognition that decision making is often based on limited time and information about a problem and that many situations are complex and rapidly changing

Boxplot: Tool in the form of a graph that displays a five-number data summary

BPR: *See* **business process reengineering**

Brainstorming: A group problem-solving technique that involves the spontaneous contribution of ideas from all members of the group

Branding communications: Messages sent to increase awareness of, and to enhance the image of, a product in the marketplace

Brand name: A patent for a new drug that gives its manufacturer the exclusive right to market the drug for a specific period of time under a brand name

Breach: A violation of a legal duty or wrongful conduct that serves as the basis for a civil remedy

Breach notification: HITECH Act Rule that requires both HIPAA-covered entities and business associates to identify unsecured PHI breaches and notify the involved parties of the breach

Breach of confidentiality: A violation of a formal or implied contract in which private information belonging to one party, but entrusted to another party, is disclosed by that individual without the consent of the party to whom the information pertains; an unauthorized disclosure of confidential information

Breach of security: A violation of security (for example, when standards of confidentiality are broken)

Break-even analysis: A financial analysis technique for determining the level of sales at which total revenues equal total costs, beyond which revenues become profits

Breast Imaging Reporting and Data System Atlas (BI-RADS): A comprehensive guide providing standardized breast imaging terminology, and a report organization, assessment structure, and a classification system for mammography, ultrasound, and MRI of the breast

Bridge technology: Technology such as document imaging and/or clinical messaging that provides some, but not all, of the benefits of an EHR

Broadband: A type of communications medium that can transmit multiple channels of data simultaneously

Browser: A program that provides a way to view and read documents available on the World Wide Web

BSC: *See* **balanced score card**

Bubble chart: A type of scatter plot with circular symbols used to compare three variables; the area of the circle indicates the value of a third variable

Budget: A plan that converts the organization's goals and objectives into targets for revenue and spending

Budget assumptions: Information about the overall organization's budget planning that sometimes includes an estimation of how revenues will increase or decrease and what limits will be placed on expenses

Budget calendar: *See* **budget cycle**

Budget cycle: The complete process of financial planning, operations, and control for a fiscal year; overlaps multiple fiscal years; *Also called* **budget calendar**

Budget neutral: 1. Adjustment of payment rates when policies change so that total spending under the new rules is the same as it would have been under the previous payment rules 2. Financial protections to ensure that overall reimbursement under the Ambulatory Payment Classification (APC) system is not greater than it would have been had the system not been in effect

Budget period: A predetermined period of time, such as a fiscal year, in which a project budget will be spent

Budget process: The process often followed from conceptualizing budget needs through working within the confines of an approved budget; *See also* **budget cycle**

Bugs: Problems in software that prevent the smooth application of a function

Buildings: A long-term (fixed) asset account that represents the physical structures owned by the organization; *See* **fixed assets**

Bundled: The grouping of Common Procedural Terminology codes related to a procedure when submitting a claim

Bundled payments: A category of payments made as lump sums to providers for all healthcare services delivered to a patient for a specific illness and/or over a specified time; a relatively continuous period in relation to a particular clinical problem or situation; they include multiple services and may include multiple providers of care; *See also* **episode-of-care reimbursement**

Bundling: Combination of supply and pharmaceutical costs or medical visits with associated procedures or services for one lump sum payment

Burden of proof: Covered entities and business associates have the burden of proof to demonstrate that all required notifications have been provided or that a use or disclosure of unsecured protected health information did not constitute a breach

Bureaucracy: A formal organizational structure based on a rigid hierarchy of decision making and inflexible rules and procedures

Bus: A type of hardware that controls the flow of commands between the central processor and other components

Business associate: 1. According to the HIPAA Privacy Rule, an individual (or group) who is not a member of a covered entity's workforce but who helps the covered entity in the performance of various functions involving the use or disclosure of individually identifiable health information 2. A person or organization other than a member of a covered entity's workforce that performs functions or activities on behalf of or affecting a covered entity that involve the use or disclosure of individually identifiable health information

Business associate agreement: A written and signed contract that allows covered entities to lawfully disclose protected health information to business associates such as consultants, billing companies, accounting firms, or others that may perform services for the provider, provided that the business associate agrees to abide by the provider's requirements to protect the information's security and confidentiality

Business case: An economic argument, or justification, usually for a capital expenditure

Business continuity plan: A program that incorporates policies and procedures for continuing business operations during a computer system shutdown; *Also called* **contingency plan; disaster planning**

Business intelligence (BI): The end product or goal of knowledge management

Business process: A set of related policies and procedures that are performed step by step to accomplish a business-related function

Business process management technology: *See* **workflow technology**

Business process reengineering (BPR): The analysis and design of the workflow within and between organizations

Business record: A record that is made and kept in the usual course of business, at or near the time of the event recorded

Business records exception: A rule under which a record is determined not to be hearsay if it was made at or near the time by, or from information transmitted by, a person with knowledge; it was kept in the course of a regularly conducted business activity; and it was the regular practice of that business activity to make the record

Business resumption: The procedure for returning a computer system to its full functionality after unscheduled downtime; similar to disaster recovery

Bylaws: Operating documents that describe the rules and regulations under which a healthcare organization operates; *See* **rules and regulations**

Bypass: Altering the route of passage of the contents of a tubular body part. Can be accomplished by rerouting contents of a body part to a downstream area of the normal route, to a similar route and body part or to an abnormal route and dissimilar body part

Byte: Eight bits treated as a single unit by a computer to represent a character

C: A high-level programming language that enables programmers to write software instructions that can be translated into machine language to run on different types of computers

C Plus Plus: An enhancement made to the original C programming language that includes classes, templates, operator overloading, and exception handling, among other improvements. C++ and C are highly compatible

CA: *See* **certificate authority**

CABG: coronary artery bypass grafting

Cache memory: A type of memory located on the central processing unit (CPU) that can also be on a part of the processor

Cafeteria plan: A health plan that allows employees to choose among two or more benefits

CAH: *See* **critical access hospital**

CAHIIM: *See* **Commission on Accreditation of Health Informatics and Information Management Education**

Calculation of inpatient service days: The measurement of the services received by all inpatients in one 24-hour period

Calculation of transfers: A medical care unit that shows transfers on and off the unit as subdivisions of patients admitted to and discharged from the unit

Calendar year (CY): Twelve-month period (year) that begins January 1 and ends December 31

Call center: A central access point to healthcare services in which clinical decision-making algorithms generate a series of questions designed to help a nurse assess a caller's healthcare condition and direct the caller to the appropriate level of service

CAM: *See* **complementary and alternative medicine; component alignment model**

CAMH: *See* **Comprehensive Accreditation Manual for Hospitals**

Cancer mortality rate: The proportion of patients that die from cancer

Cancer registry: Records maintained by many states for the purpose of tracking the incidence (new cases) of cancer

Cap: *See* **capitation**

CAP: *See* **College of American Pathologists**; **corrective action plan**

Capital assets: Physical assets with an estimated useful life of more than one year; *See* **fixed assets**; **property, plant, and equipment (PPE)**

Capital budget: The allocation of resources for long-term investments and projects

Capital budget process: A four-stage process organizations follow to determine what capital projects to include in the budget

Capitated patient: A patient enrolled in a managed care program that pays a fixed monthly payment to the patient's identified primary care provider

Capitated payment: A managed care term that refers to the fixed amount a physician or other healthcare provider is paid to provide services to a patient or a group of patients over a prespecified period of time

Capitation: A method of healthcare reimbursement in which an insurance carrier prepays a physician, hospital, or other healthcare provider a fixed amount for a given population without regard to the actual number or nature of healthcare services provided to the population

CAQH: *See* **Council for Affordable Quality Healthcare**

Care: The management of, responsibility for, or attention to the safety and well-being of other persons in the context of healthcare settings

Career development: The process of growing or progressing within one's profession or occupation

Career planning: Looking beyond simply getting a job to position oneself for more challenging and diverse work in the long term

Caregiver: 1. Any clinical professional (physician, nurse, technologist, or therapist, for example) who provides care directly to patients 2. A nonprofessional who provides supportive assistance in a residential setting to a relative, friend, or client who is seriously ill

Care Map®: A proprietary care-planning tool similar to a clinical protocol that outlines the major aspects of treatment on the basis of diagnosis or other characteristics of the patient

Care path: A care-planning tool similar to a clinical practice guideline that has a multidisciplinary focus emphasizing the coordination of clinical services; *Also called* **clinical algorithm**; *See* **clinical pathway**; **critical path or critical pathway**

Care plan: The specific goals in the treatment of an individual patient, amended as the patient's condition requires, and the assessment of the outcomes of care; serves as the primary source for ongoing documentation of the resident's care, condition, and needs

Care planning: The process of organizing and documenting the specific goals in the treatment of an individual patient, amending the goals as the patient's condition requires, and assessing the outcomes of care

Care unit: An organizational entity of a healthcare facility; healthcare facilities are organized both physically and functionally into units to provide care

CARF: *See* **Commission on Accreditation of Rehabilitation Facilities**

Carrier: 1. The insurance company; the insurer that sold the policy and administers the benefits 2. Entity that has a contract with the Centers for Medicare and Medicaid Services (CMS) to determine and make Medicare payments for Part B benefits

Carrier, Medicare: An organization under contract with the Centers for Medicare and Medicaid Services to serve as the financial agent that works with providers and the federal government to locally administer Medicare eligibility and payments

Carriers (Medicare Part B): Financial agents that serve under contract with the Centers for Medicare and Medicaid Services to work with providers and the federal government to locally administer Medicare Part B claims

Carve-outs: Applicable services that are cut out of the contract and paid at a different rate

Case: Patient, resident, or client with a given condition or disease

Case-based payment: Type of prospective payment method in which the third-party payer reimburses the provider a fixed, preestablished payment for each case

Case-control study: A study that investigates the development of disease by amassing volumes of data about factors in the lives of persons with the disease (cases) and persons without the disease; *See* **retrospective study**

Case definition: A method of determining criteria for cases that should be included in a registry

Case fatality rate: The total number of deaths due to a specific illness during a given time period divided by the total number of cases during the same period

Case finding: A method of identifying patients who have been seen and/or treated in a healthcare facility for the particular disease or condition of interest to the registry

Case law: *See* **common law**

Case management: 1. The ongoing, concurrent review performed by clinical professionals to ensure the necessity and effectiveness of the clinical services being provided to a patient 2. A process that integrates and coordinates patient care over time and across multiple sites and providers, especially in complex and high-cost cases, with goals of continuity of care, cost-effectiveness, quality, and appropriate utilization 3. The process of developing a specific care plan for a patient that serves as a communication tool to improve quality of care and reduce cost

Case management services: Services in which a physician is responsible for direct care of a patient, as well as for coordinating and controlling access to, or initiating and/or supervising other healthcare services for, the patient

Case manager: 1. A professional nurse who coordinates the daily progress of a patient population by assessing needs, developing goals, individualizing plans of care on an ongoing basis, and evaluating overall progress 2. A medical professional (usually a nurse or a social worker) who reviews cases to determine the necessity of care and to advise providers on payer's utilization restrictions

Case mix: 1. A description of a patient population based on any number of specific characteristics, including age, gender, type of insurance, diagnosis, risk factors, treatment received, and resources used 2. Set of categories of patients (type and volume) treated by a healthcare organization and representing the complexity of the organization's caseload

Case-mix group (CMG) relative weights: Factors that account for the variance in cost per discharge and resource utilization among case-mix groups

Case-mix groups (CMGs): The 97 function-related groups into which inpatient rehabilitation facility discharges are classified on the basis of the patient's level of impairment, age, comorbidities, functional ability, and other factors

Case-mix index (CMI): The average relative weight of all cases treated at a given facility or by a given physician, which reflects the resource intensity or clinical severity of a specific group in relation to the other groups in the classification system; calculated by dividing the sum of the weights of diagnosis-related groups for patients discharged during a given period by the total number of patients discharged

Case-mix system: A system for grouping cases that are clinically similar and ordinarily consume similar resources; used to provide information about the types of patients treated by a facility

Case study: A type of nonparticipant observation in which researchers investigate one person, one group, or one institution in depth

Cash: The actual money that has been received and is readily available to pay debts; a short-term (current) asset account that represents currency and bank account balances; *See* **current asset**

Cash accounting: A method of accounting that is used most frequently in a sole proprietorship or a small business environment that recognizes income and expense transactions when cash is received or cash is paid out

Cash budget: A forecast of needs for available funds throughout the year

Cash conversion cycle: The period that refers to expenditures needed to provide services to patients through the reimbursement or collection of fees for those provided services

Cash flow: The availability of money to pay the organization's bills (receipts minus disbursements)

Catastrophic coverage: *See* **major medical insurance**

Catastrophic expense limit: Specific amount, in a certain time frame such as one year, beyond which all covered healthcare services for that policyholder or dependent are paid at 100 percent by the healthcare insurance plan; *See* **maximum out-of-pocket cost**; **stop-loss benefit**

Categorical data: Four types of data (nominal, ordinal, interval, and ratio) that represent values or observations that can be sorted into a category; *See* **scales of measurement**

Categorically needy eligibility groups: Categories of individuals to whom states must provide coverage under the federal Medicaid program

Category I codes: Procedures or services identified by a five-digit CPT code and organized within the six sections

Category II codes: CPT codes that describe services or test results that are agreed upon as contributing to positive health outcomes and high-quality patient care. They are for performance measurement, and use of these codes is optional

Category III codes: CPT codes that describe new and emerging technology. They may be published at any time during the year, rather than on the annual publication cycle, and can be found on the AMA website (www.ama-assn.org) and immediately preceding the alphabetic index in the CPT codebook

Causal-comparative research: A research design that resembles experimental research but lacks random assignment to a group and manipulation of treatment; *Also called* **quasi experimental design**

Causal relationship: A type of relationship in which one factor results in a change in another factor (cause and effect)

Causation: In law, a relationship between the defendant's conduct and the harm that was suffered

Cause-and-effect diagram: An investigational technique that facilitates the identification of the various factors that contribute to a problem; *See* **fishbone diagram**

Cause-specific death rate: The total number of deaths due to a specific illness during a given time period divided by the estimated population for the same time period

CBSA: *See* **core-based statistical area**

CC: *See* **chief complaint; complications/comorbidities**

CCA: Certified coding associate

CCC: *See* **Clinical Care Classification**

CCD: *See* **Continuity of Care Document**

CCHIT: *See* **Certification Commission on Health Information Technology**

CCI: *See* Correct Coding Initiative

CCOW: *See* Clinical Context Object Workgroup

CCR: *See* Continuity of Care Record

CCS: *See* certified coding specialist

CCS-P: *See* certified coding specialist–physician based

CCU: *See* cardiac care unit; coronary care unit

CD: *See* compact disc

CDA: *See* Clinical Document Architecture

CDC: *See* Centers for Disease Control and Prevention

CDER Manual: *See* Center for Drug Evaluation and Research Data Standards Manual

CDHP: *See* consumer-directed (driven) healthcare plan

CDI: *See* clinical documentation improvement

CDM: *See* charge description master

CDR: *See* clinical data repository

CDS: *See* clinical decision support

CDSS: *See* clinical decision support system

CDT: *See* Current Dental Terminology

CDW: *See* clinical data warehouse

CE: *See* covered entity

CEN: *See* European Committee for Standardization

Census: The number of inpatients present in a healthcare facility at any given time

Census day: *See* inpatient service day

Census-reporting policy: A policy that outlines the process for census reporting and tracking

Census statistics: Statistics that examine the number of patients being treated at specific times, the length of their stay, and the number of times a bed changes occupants

Census survey: A survey that collects data from all the members of a population

Center of Excellence: A healthcare facility selected to provide specific services based on criteria such as experience, outcomes, efficiency, and effectiveness. Tertiary and academic medical centers are often designated as centers of excellence for one or more services such as organ transplantation

Center for Drug Evaluation and Research (CDER) Data Standards Manual: A compilation of standardized nomenclature monographs for sharing information regarding manufactured drug dosage forms

Centers for Disease Control and Prevention (CDC): A group of federal agencies that oversee health promotion and disease control and prevention activities in the United States

Centers for Medicare and Medicaid Services (CMS): The division of the Department of Health and Human Services that is responsible for developing healthcare policy in the United States and for administering the Medicare program and the federal portion of the Medicaid program and maintaining the procedure portion of the International Classification of Diseases, ninth revision, Clinical Modification (ICD-9-CM); called the Health Care Financing Administration (HCFA) prior to 2001

Central data repository: *See* **data repository**

Central processing unit: The brain of a computer, or the circuits that make the electrical parts function

Central tendency: A statistical term referring to the center of the distribution; an average or middle value

CEO: *See* **chief executive officer**

Certainty factor: The defined certainty percentage rate with which an occurrence must present itself to satisfy quality standards

Certificate holder: Member of a group for which an employer or association has purchased group healthcare insurance; *See* **insured member**; **policyholder**; **subscriber**

Certificate of coverage: A written description of benefits included in a health plan and required by state law

Certificate of destruction: A document that constitutes proof that a health record was destroyed and that includes the method of destruction, the signature of the person responsible for destruction, and inclusive dates for destruction

Certificate of need (CON): A state-directed program that requires healthcare facilities to submit detailed plans and justifications for the purchase of new equipment, new buildings, or new service offerings that cost in excess of a certain amount

Certification: 1. The process by which a duly authorized body evaluates and recognizes an individual, institution, or educational program as meeting predetermined requirements 2. An evaluation performed to establish the extent to which a particular computer system, network design, or application implementation meets a prespecified set of requirements

Certification authority (CA): An independent licensing agency that vouches for a person's identity in encrypted electronic communications

Certification Commission for Healthcare Information Technology (CCHIT): An independent, voluntary, private-sector initiative organized as a limited liability corporation that has been awarded a contract by the US Department of Health and Human Services (HHS) to develop, create prototypes for, and evaluate the certification criteria and inspection process for electronic health record products (EHRs)

Certified Guidance Document (CGD): Under ARRA, the purpose is to explain the factors ONC will use to determine whether or not to recommend to the Secretary of HHS a body as a Recommended Certification Body (RCB). The CGD will serve as a guide for ONC as it evaluates applications for RCB status and seeks to provide all of the information a body would need to apply for and obtain such status

Certification/recertification: Medicare requirement for the physician's official recognition of skilled nursing care needs for the resident

Certification standards: Detailed compulsory requirements for participation in Medicare and Medicaid programs

Certified coding associate (CCA): An AHIMA credential awarded to entry-level coders who have demonstrated skill in classifying medical data by passing a certification exam

Certified coding specialist (CCS): An AHIMA credential awarded to individuals who have demonstrated skill in classifying medical data from patient records, generally in the hospital setting, by passing a certification examination

Certified coding specialist—physician based (CCS–P) An AHIMA credential awarded to individuals who have demonstrated coding expertise in physician-based settings, such as group practices, by passing a certification examination

Certified EHR Technology: 1. A Complete EHR that meets the requirements included in the definition of a Qualified EHR and has been tested and certified in accordance with the certification program established by the National Coordinator as having met all applicable certification criteria adopted by the Secretary 2. A combination of EHR modules in which each constituent EHR module of the combination has been tested and certified in accordance with the certification program established by the National Coordinator as having met all applicable certification criteria adopted by the Secretary, and the resultant combination also meets the requirements included in the definition of a Qualified EHR

Certified health data analyst (CHDA): An AHIMA credential awarded to individuals who have demonstrated skills and expertise in health data analysis

Certified Information Systems Security Professional (CISSP): Certification sponsored by the International Information Systems Security Certification Consortium (ISC); it is a generic security certification and therefore is not healthcare specific

Certified in healthcare privacy (CHP): AHIMA credential denoting advanced competency in designing, implementing, and administering comprehensive privacy protection programs in all types of healthcare organizations; requires baccalaureate or master's degree, or healthcare information management credential plus experience

Certified in healthcare privacy and security (CHPS): AHIMA credential that recognizes advanced competency in designing, implementing, and administering comprehensive privacy and security protection programs in all types of healthcare organizations; requires successful completion of the CHPS exam sponsored by AHIMA

Certified in healthcare security (CHS): Credential (managed by HIMSS) that certifies advanced abilities in designing, implementing, and administering comprehensive security programs

Certified medical transcriptionist (CMT): A certification that is granted upon successfully passing the Association of Healthcare Documentation Integrity (AHDI) certification examination for medical transcriptionists with generally at least two years of experience

Certified nurse-midwife (CNM): An individual trained in the dual disciplines of nursing and midwifery who has successfully completed an accredited program of study and clinical experience in nurse-midwifery. They are certified according to the requirements of the American College of Nurse-Midwives

Certified professional coder (CPC): Credential sponsored by the American Academy of Professional Coders that certifies physician coders

Certified professional coder-hospital (CPC-H): Credential sponsored by the American Academy of Professional Coders that certifies hospital-based coders

Certified professional in health information management systems (CPHIMS): Credential (managed jointly by HIMSS, AHA Certification Center, and applied measurement professionals) that certifies knowledge of healthcare information and management systems and understanding of psychometrics (the science of measurement); requires baccalaureate or graduate degree plus associated experience

Certified public accountant (CPA): An individual who has achieved specialized expertise in using and managing financial accounting information

Certified Registered Nurse Anesthetist (CRNA): A registered nurse who has completed additional training in anesthesia and provides anesthesia for a wide variety of surgical cases

Cesarean section rate: The ratio of all cesarean sections to the total number of deliveries, including cesarean sections, during a specified period of time

CF: *See* **conversion factor; national conversation factor**

CFO: *See* **chief financial officer**

CFR: *See* **Code of Federal Regulations**

CGD: *See* **Certified Guidance Document**

Chain of command: A hierarchical reporting structure within an organization

Chain of trust: In the HIPAA Security Rule, a requirement that each covered entity that shares healthcare data with another entity requires that the entity provide protections comparable to those provided by the covered entity

Champion: An individual within an organization who believes in an innovation or change and promotes the idea by building financial and political support

CHAMPUS: *See* **Civilian Health and Medical Program–Uniformed Services**

CHAMPVA: *See* **Civilian Health and Medical Program–Veterans Administration**

Change: Under ICD-10-PCS, a root procedure defined as taking out or off a device from a body part and putting back an identical or similar device in or on the same body part without cutting or puncturing the skin or a mucous membrane. Represents only those procedures where a similar device is exchanged without making a new incision or puncture

Change agent: An individual within an organization whose primary responsibility is to facilitate change

Change control: The process of performing an impact analysis and obtaining approval before modifications to the project scope are made

Change drivers: Forces in the external environment of organizations or industries that force organizations or industries to change the way they operate in order to survive

Change management: The formal process of introducing change, getting it adopted, and diffusing it throughout the organization

CHAP: *See* **Community Health Accreditation Program**

Charge: In healthcare, a price assigned to a unit of medical or health service, such as a visit to a physician or a day in a hospital; may be unrelated to the actual cost of providing the service; *See* **fee**

Charge capture: The process of collecting all services, procedures, and supplies provided during patient care

Charge code: The numerical identification of a service or supply that links the item to a particular department within the charge description master

Charge description master (CDM): *See* **chargemaster**

Charge entry: The act of entering ICD-9-CM, CPT, or HCPCS codes into a computerized billing system for services provided during a patient visit or procedure. In the EHR, this process occurs automatically

Charge reconciliation: The act of reviewing charges entered for claims submission by the charge entry process. Ensures that all services, procedures, and supplies are available and pass to the claim form

Chargemaster: A financial management form that contains information about the organization's charges for the healthcare services it provides to patients; *Also called* **charge description master (CDM)**

Charges: The dollar amounts actually billed by healthcare facilities for specific services or supplies and owed by patients

Charge ticket: The tool used to collect data for the billing process; *Also called* billing slip; charge slip; encounter form; fee slip; fee ticket; route slip; route tag; superbill

Charisma: The ability of a leader to inspire and motivate others to high performance and commitment

Charitable immunity: A doctrine that shielded hospitals (as well as other institutions) from liability for negligence because of the belief that donors would not make contributions to hospitals if they thought their donation would be used to litigate claims combined with concern that a few lawsuits could bankrupt a hospital

Charity care: Services for which healthcare organizations did not expect payment because they had previously determined the patients' or clients' inability to pay

Chart: 1. (noun) The health record of a patient 2. (verb) To document information about a patient in a health record

Chart conversion: An EHR implementation activity in which data from the paper chart are converted into electronic form

Chart deficiency system: A software system designed to allow the HIM department to electronically track and manage documentation omissions from the health record

Chart locator system: A software system designed to track the location of paper health records as they are viewed by healthcare professionals, for example, a record checked to quality management for review

Chart order policy: A policy that provides a detailed listing of all documents and defines their order and section location within the health record

Chart tracking: A process that identifies the current location of a paper record or information

Chart-tracking/requests policy: A policy that outlines the way in which charts are signed out of the permanent files and how requests for records are handled

Charting by exception: A system of health record documentation in which progress notes focus on abnormal events and describe any interventions that were ordered and the patient's response; *Also called* focus charting

CHD: *See* **community health dimension**

CHDA: *See* **Certified Health Data Analyst** ordered and the patient's response; *Also called* **focus charting**

Check digit: A representation of a checksum operation

Checksheet: A tool that permits the systematic recording of observations of a particular phenomenon so that trends or patterns can be identified

Checksum: Digits or bits summed according to arbitrary rules and used to verify the integrity of numerical data

Cherry picking: In reimbursement, the term given when payers target the enrollment of healthy patients to minimize healthcare costs

CHI: *See* **Consolidated Health Informatics**

Chief complaint: The principal problem a patient reports to a healthcare provider

Chief executive officer (CEO): The senior manager appointed by a governing board to direct an organization's overall long-term strategic management

Chief financial officer (CFO): The senior manager responsible for the fiscal management of an organization

Chief information officer (CIO): The senior manager responsible for the overall management of information resources in an organization

Chief information security officer (CISO): IT leadership role responsible for overseeing the development, implementation, and enforcement of a healthcare organization's security program; role has grown as a direct result of the HIPAA security regulations

Chief information technology officer (CITO): IT leadership role that guides an organization's decisions related to technical architecture and evaluates the latest technology developments and their applicability or potential use in the organization

Chief knowledge officer (CKO): A position that oversees the entire knowledge acquisition, storage, and dissemination process and that identifies subject matter experts to help capture and organize the organization's knowledge assets

Chief medical informatics officer (CMIO): An emerging position, typically a physician with medical informatics training, that provides physician leadership and direction in the deployment of clinical applications in healthcare organizations

Chief nursing officer (CNO): The senior manager (usually a registered nurse with advanced education and extensive experience) responsible for administering patient care services

Chief of staff: The physician designated as leader of a healthcare organization's medical staff

Chief operating officer (COO): An executive-level role responsible at a high level for day-to-day operations of an organization

Chief privacy officer: A position that oversees activities related to the development, implementation, and maintenance of, and adherence to, organizational policies and procedures regarding the privacy of and access to patient-specific information and ensures compliance with federal and state laws and regulations and accrediting body standards concerning the confidentiality and privacy of health-related information

Chief security officer (CSO): The middle manager responsible for overseeing all aspects of an organization's security plan

Children's Health Insurance Program (CHIP): *See* **State Children's Health Insurance Program (SCHIP)**

Child Welfare League of America (CWLA): An association of public and private nonprofit agencies and organizations across the United States and Canada devoted to improving life for abused, neglected, and otherwise vulnerable children and young people and their families

CHIME: *See* **College of Health Information Management Executives**

CHIN: *See* **community health information network**

CHIP: *See* **Children's Health Insurance Program**

Chi-square: A statistical calculation used to determine whether proportions in a randomly drawn sample are significantly different from the underlying or theoretical population proportions

CHP: *See* **certified in healthcare privacy**

CHPS: *See* **certified healthcare privacy and security**

Chronic: Used when specifying a medical disease or illness of long duration

Chronological order: A method of sequencing the health record according to time where the most recent document is found at the end of the health record

CHS: *See* **certified in healthcare security**

CIA: *See* **Corporate Integrity Agreement**

CIO: *See* **chief information officer**

Cipher text: A text message that has been encrypted, or converted into code, to make it unreadable in order to conceal its meaning

Circuit: The geographic area covered by a US Court of Appeals

Circuit courts: Federal appellate courts distributed through the United States, including the District of Columbia and US territories, so that each court represents a specific number of the district courts

Circumstantial evidence: A form of evidence that is not directly from an eyewitness or participant and requires some reasoning to prove a fact

Circuit switching: Communications technology that establishes a connection between callers in a telephone network using a dedicated circuit path

CIS: *See* **clinical information system**

CISO: *See* **chief information security officer**

CISSP: *See* **Certified Information Systems Security Professional**

CITO: *See* **chief information technology officer**

Civilian Health and Medical Program—Uniformed Services (CHAMPUS): A federal program providing supplementary civilian-sector hospital and medical services beyond that which is available in military treatment facilities to military dependents, retirees and their dependents, and certain others

Civilian Health and Medical Program—Veterans Administration (CHAMPVA): The federal healthcare benefits program for dependents (spouse or widow[er] and children) of veterans rated by the Veterans Administration (VA) as having a total and permanent disability, for survivors of veterans who died from VA-rated service-connected conditions or who were rated permanently and totally disabled at the time of death from a VA-rated service-connected condition, and for survivors of persons who died in the line of duty

Civil law: The branch of law involving court actions among private parties, corporations, government bodies, or other organizations, typically for the recovery of private rights with compensation usually being monetary

Civil Monetary Penalties Act (CMP): Section 1128A of the Social Security Act, passed in 1981 as one of several administrative remedies to combat increases in health-care fraud and abuse, which authorized the Secretary and Inspector General of Health and Human Services (HHS) to impose civil monetary penalties, assessment, and program exclusions on individuals and entities whose wrongdoing caused injury to HHS programs or their beneficiaries

Civil procedure: The rules and parameters that govern civil (noncriminal) cases

Civil proceeding (action): An action brought to enforce, redress, or protect private rights or to protect a private right or compel a civil remedy in a dispute between private parties (in general, all types of actions other than criminal proceedings)

Civil Rights Act of 1991: The federal legislation that focuses on establishing an employer's responsibility for justifying hiring practices that seem to adversely affect people because of race, color, religion, sex, or national origin

Civil Rights Act, Title VII (1964): The federal legislation that prohibits discrimination in employment on the basis of race, religion, color, sex, or national origin

CKO: *See* **chief knowledge officer**

Claim: An itemized statement of healthcare services and their costs provided by a hospital, physician office, or other healthcare provider; submitted for reimbursement to the healthcare insurance plan by either the insured party or by the provider

Claim adjustment reason codes: A national administrative code set, used in X12 835 and X12 837 Claim Payment and Remittance Advice and Claims Transactions, that identifies the reasons for any differences or adjustments between the original provider charge for a claim or service and the payer's payment for it

Claim attachment: Any of a variety of hardcopy or electronic forms needed to process a claim in addition to the claim itself, such as a copy of the emergency department note

Claim status code: A national administrative code set, identified in X12 277 Claims Status Notification transactions, that identifies the status of healthcare claims

Claims management: A function related to risk management that enables an organization to track descriptive claims information (incidents, claimants, insurance, demands, dates, and so on), along with data on investigation, litigation, settlement, defendants, and subrogation

Claims processing: The process of accumulating claims for services, submitting claims for reimbursement, and ensuring that claims are satisfied

Claims scrubber software: A type of computer program at a healthcare facility that checks the claim elements for accuracy and agreement before the claims are submitted

Class: The higher-level abstraction of an object that defines its properties and operations

Classification: A clinical vocabulary, terminology, or nomenclature that lists words or phrases with their meanings, provides for the proper use of clinical words as names or symbols, and facilitates mapping standardized terms to broader classifications for administrative, regulatory, oversight, and fiscal requirements

Classification system: 1. A system for grouping similar diseases and procedures and organizing related information for easy retrieval 2. A system for assigning numeric or alphanumeric code numbers to represent specific diseases and/or procedures

Clean claim: A completed insurance claim form that contains all the required information (without any missing information) so that it can be processed and paid promptly

Clearinghouse: *See* **Healthcare clearinghouse**

CLIA: *See* **Clinical Laboratory Improvement Amendments**

Client: A patient who receives behavioral or mental health services

Client/server architecture: A computer architecture in which multiple computers (clients) are connected to other computers (servers) that store and distribute large amounts of shared data

Clinic: An outpatient facility providing a limited range of healthcare services and assuming overall healthcare responsibility for patients

Clinical abstract: A computerized file that summarizes patient demographics and other information, including reason for admission, diagnoses, procedures, physician information, and any additional information deemed pertinent by the facility

Clinical algorithm: *See* **care path**

Clinical Care Classification (CCC): Two interrelated taxonomies, the CCC of Nursing Diagnoses and Outcomes and the CCC of Nursing Interventions and Actions, that provide a standardized framework for documenting patient care in hospitals, home health agencies, ambulatory care clinics, and other healthcare settings

Clinical care plans: Care guidelines created by healthcare providers for individual patients for a specified period of time

Clinical coding: The process of assigning numeric or alphanumeric classifications to diagnostic and procedural statements

Clinical communication space: The context and range of electronic and interpersonal information exchanged among staff and patients

Clinical Context Object Workgroup (CCOW): A standard protocol developed by HL7 to allow clinical applications to share information at the point of care

Clinical data: Data captured during the process of diagnosis and treatment

Clinical data manager: The person responsible for managing the data collected during the research project, developing data standards, conducting clinical coding for specific data elements, determining the best database to house the data, choosing appropriate software systems to analyze the data, and conducting data entry and data analysis; includes various responsibilities according to the research study protocol

Clinical data repository (CDR): A central database that focuses on clinical information

Clinical data warehouse (CDW): A database that makes it possible to access data from multiple databases and combine the results into a single query and reporting interface; *See also* **data warehouse**

Clinical decision support (CDS): The process in which individual data elements are represented in the computer by a special code to be used in making comparisons, trending results, and supplying clinical reminders and alerts

Clinical decision support system (CDSS): A special subcategory of clinical information systems that is designed to help healthcare providers make knowledge-based clinical decisions

Clinical Document Architecture (CDA): An HL7 XML-based document markup standard for the electronic exchange model for clinical documents (such as discharge summaries and progress notes)

Clinical documentation: Any manual or electronic notation (or recording) made by a physician or other healthcare clinician related to a patient's medical condition or treatment

Clinical Documentation Improvement (CDI): The process an organization undertakes that will improve clinical specificity and documentation that will allow coders to assign more concise disease classification codes

Clinical Documentation Improvement Plan (CDIP): A program in which specialists concurrently review health records for incomplete documentation, prompting clinical staff to clarify ambiguity which allows coders to assign more concise disease classification codes

Clinical documentation system: *See* **clinical decision support (CDS)**

Clinical domain: A domain that captures significant indicators of clinical needs from several OASIS items, including patient history and sensory, integumentary, respiratory, elimination, neurological, emotional, and behavioral status

Clinical drug: A pharmaceutical product given to (or taken by) a patient with a therapeutic or diagnostic intent; it has a clinical drug name, which includes the routed generic, the strength, and dose form

Clinical guidelines/protocols: With clinical care plans and clinical pathways, a predetermined method of performing healthcare for a specific disease or other clinical situation based on clinical evidence that the method provides high-quality, cost-effective healthcare; *Also called* **treatment guidelines/protocols**

Clinical informatics: A field of information science concerned with the management of data and information used to support the practice and delivery of patient care through the application of computers and computer technologies

Clinical information: Health record documentation that describes the patient's condition and course of treatment

Clinical information system (CIS): A category of a health-care information system that includes systems that directly support patient care

Clinical integration: The operational integration of a variety of healthcare services from the same health-care organization with the purpose of streamlining administrative processes and increasing potential for improved clinical outcomes for the benefit of the patient

Clinical Laboratory Improvement Amendments (CLIA): Passed in 1988, the amendments established quality standards for all laboratory testing to ensure the accuracy, reliability, and timeliness of patient test results regardless of where the test is

Clinical/medical decision support system: A data-driven decision support system that assists physicians in applying new information to patient care through the analysis of patient-specific clinical and medical variables

Clinical messaging: The function of electronically delivering data and automating the workflow around the management of clinical data

Clinical pathway: A tool designed to coordinate multidisciplinary care planning for specific diagnoses and treatments; *See* **Care Map®**; **critical path**

Clinical pertinence review: A review of medical records performed to assess the quality of information using criteria determined by the healthcare organization; includes quantitative and qualitative components

Clinical practice guidelines: A detailed, step-by-step guide used by healthcare practitioners to make knowledge-based decisions related to patient care and issued by an authoritative organization such as a medical society or government agency; *See* **clinical protocol**

Clinical practice standards: The established criteria against which the decisions and actions of healthcare practitioners and other representatives of healthcare organizations are assessed in accordance with state and federal laws, regulations, and guidelines; the codes of ethics published by professional associations or societies; the criteria for accreditation published by accreditation agencies; or the usual and common practice of similar clinicians or organizations in a geographical region

Clinical privileges: The authorization granted by a health-care organization's governing board to a member of the medical staff that enables the physician to provide patient services in the organization within specific practice limits

Clinical protocol: Specific instructions for performing clinical procedures established by authoritative bodies, such as medical staff committees, and intended to be applied literally and universally; *See* **clinical practice guidelines**

Clinical provider order entry: *See* **computerized provider order entry**

Clinical quality assessment: The process for determining whether the services provided to patients meet prede-termined standards of care

Clinical repository: A frequently updated database that pro-vides users with direct access to detailed patient-level data as well as the ability to drill down into historical views of administrative, clinical, and financial data; *Also called* **data warehouse**

Clinical research: A specialized area of research that pri-marily investigates the efficacy of preventive, diagnos-tic, and therapeutic procedures; *Also called* **medical research**

Clinical research associate: A person who develops new study protocols; hires investigators; writes progress reports, data and safety monitoring plans, and subse-quent reports of any adverse events; and takes part in writing publications upon completion of the project

Clinical research coordinator: The person who runs the research project and ensures that the clinical protocol is followed as written

Clinical risk group (CRG): Capitated prospective payment system that predicts future healthcare expenditures for populations

Clinical service: A general term used to indicate a unit of medical staff responsibility (such as cardiology), a unit of inpatient beds (such as general medicine), or even a group of discharged patients with related diseases or treatment (such as orthopedic)

Clinical Special Product Label (SPL): A LOINC standard that provides information found in the approved FDA drug label or package insert in a computer-readable format for use in electronic prescribing and decision support

Clinical systems: Applications that focus on supporting documentation, information retrieval, and knowledge generation at the point of care by providers, that is, physicians, nurses, therapists, pharmacists, and others

Clinical systems analyst: *See* **systems analyst**

Clinical terminology: A set of standardized terms and their synonyms that record patient findings, circumstances, events, and interventions with sufficient detail to support clinical care, decision support, outcomes research, and quality improvement; *See* **nomenclature**

Clinical Terms, Version 3 (CTV3): A crown copyright work of the National Health Service in the United Kingdom that comprises a coded terminology designed to facilitate the exchange, retrieval, and analysis of key data in the medical record; formerly known as the Read Codes

Clinical trial: 1. A controlled research study involving human subjects that is designed to evaluate prospectively the safety and effectiveness of new drugs, tests, devices, or interventions 2. Experimental study in which an intervention or treatment is given to one group in a clinical setting and the outcomes compared with a control group that did not have the intervention or treatment or that had a different intervention or treatment

Clinical value compass: Performance improvement approach that measures the association of quality and value

Clinical vocabulary: A formally recognized list of preferred medical terms; *Also called* **medical vocabulary**

Clinical vocabulary manager: A role within an organization that manages classification systems and vocabularies for the organization

Clinical workstation: A single point of access that includes a common user interface to view information from disparate applications and to launch applications

Clinician: A healthcare provider, including physicians and others who treat patients

Clinician/physician web portals: The media for providing physician/clinician access to the provider organization's multiple sources of data from any network-connected device

Clinic outpatient: A patient who is admitted to a clinical service of a clinic or hospital for diagnosis or treatment on an ambulatory basis

Clinic referral: *See* **source of admission**

Clinic without walls (CWW): *See* **group practice without walls**

Closed-ended question: *See* **structured question**

Closed panel: Type of health maintenance organization that provides hospitalization and physicians' services through its own staff and facilities; beneficiaries are allowed to use only those specified facilities and physicians or dentists who accept the plan or organization's conditions of membership and reimbursement; *See* **group model health maintenance organization**; **staff model health maintenance organization**

Closed-record review: A review of records after a patient has been discharged from the organization or treatment has been terminated

Closed record: 1. A health record that has been closed following analysis to ensure all documentation components are met, for example, signatures and dictated reports 2. Documentation or a note that has been closed due to system requirements or after a defined period of time

Closed systems: Systems that operate in a self-contained environment

Clustering: The practice of coding/charging one or two middle levels of service codes exclusively, under the philosophy that some will be higher, some lower, and the charges will average out over an extended period

Cluster sampling: The process of selecting subjects for a sample from each cluster within a population (for example, a family, school, or community)

CME: *See* **Continuing medical education**

CMG: *See* **case-mix groups**

CMI: *See* **case-mix index**

CMIO: *See* **chief medical informatics officer**

CMP: *See* **Civil Monetary Penalties Act**

CMS: *See* **Centers for Medicare and Medicaid Services**

CMS-485: A Medicare form used to document care plans

CMS-1450: A Medicare form used for standardized uniform billing for hospital services

CMS-1500: 1. The universal insurance claim form developed and approved by the American Medical Association (AMA) and the Centers for Medicare and Medicaid Services (CMS) that physicians use to bill Medicare, Medicaid, and private insurers for professional services provided 2. A Medicare claim form used to bill third-party payers for provider services, for example, physician office visits

CMT: *See* **certified medical transcriptionist**; also, chiropractic manipulative treatment

CNM: *See* **certified nurse-midwife**

CNO: *See* **chief nursing officer**

CNS: central nervous system

COA: *See* **Council on Accreditation**

Coaching: 1. A training method in which an experienced person gives advice to a less-experienced worker on a formal or informal basis 2. A disciplinary method used as the first step for employees who are not meeting performance expectations

Coalition building: A technique used to manage the political dimensions of change within an organization by building the support of groups for change

COBRA: *See* **Consolidated Omnibus Budget Reconciliation Act of 1975**

COB: *See* **coordination of benefits**

COB transaction: *See* **coordination of benefits transaction**

CoC: *See* **Commission on Cancer**

Code: In information systems, software instructions that direct computers to perform a specified action; in healthcare, an alphanumeric representation of the terms in a clinical classification or vocabulary

Coded data: Data that are translated into a standard nomenclature of classification so that they may be aggregated, analyzed, and compared

Code edit: An accuracy checkpoint in the claims-processing software, such as female procedures done only on female patients

Code editor: Software that evaluates the clinical consistency and completeness of health record information and identifies potential errors that could affect accurate prospective payment group assignment

Code lookup: A computer file with all of the indexes and codes recorded on magnetic disk or CD-ROM

Code of ethics: A statement of ethical principles regarding business practices and professional behavior

Code of Federal Regulations (CFR): The official collection of legislative and regulatory guidelines mandated by final rules published in the *Federal Register*

Coder: A person assigned solely to the function of coding

Code range: Applicable set of diagnosis or procedure codes

Coder/biller: A person in an ambulatory care or a physician office setting who is generally responsible for processing the superbill

Code Set: Under HIPAA, any set of codes used to encode data elements, such as tables of terms, medical concepts, medical diagnostic codes, or medical procedure codes; includes both the codes and their descriptions

Code Set Maintenance Organization: 1. Under HIPAA, the organization that creates and maintains the code sets adopted by the Secretary of HHS for use in the transactions for which standards are adopted 2. Part II, 45 CFR 162.103

Coding: The process of assigning numeric or alphanumeric representations to clinical documentation

Coding Clinic for HCPCS: A publication issued quarterly by the American Hospital Association and approved by the Centers for Medicare and Medicaid Services to give coding advice and direction for HCPCS code assignment

Coding Clinic for ICD-9-CM: A publication issued quarterly by the American Hospital Association and approved by the Centers for Medicare and Medicaid Services to give coding advice and direction for ICD-9-CM

Coding compliance plan: A component of an HIM compliance plan or a corporate compliance plan modeling the OIG Program Guidance for Hospitals and the OIG Supplemental Compliance Program Guidance for Hospitals that focuses on the unique regulations and guidelines with which coding professionals must comply

Coding formalization principles: A set of principles referring to the transition of coding from analysis of records to a process that involves data analysis using more sophisticated tools (for example, algorithmic translation, concept representation, or vocabulary or reimbursement mapping)

Coding specialist: The healthcare worker responsible for assigning numeric or alphanumeric codes to diagnostic or procedural statements

Cognitive: Related to mental abilities, such as talking, memory, and problem solving

Cohort study: A study, followed over time, in which a group of subjects is identified as having one or more characteristics in common

Coinsurance: Cost sharing in which the policy or certificate holder pays a preestablished percentage of eligible expenses after the deductible has been met; the percentage may vary by type or site of service

COLA: *See* **cost-of-living adjustment**

COLD/ERM: *See* **computer output to laser disk/enterprise report management**

Cold site: In disaster planning, a basic facility with adequate space and infrastructure (electrical power, telecommunications) to support the organization's information systems

Collaborative Stage Data Set: A new standardized neoplasm-staging system developed by the American Joint Commission on Cancer

Collection: 1. The part of the billing process in which payment for services performed is obtained 2. In AHIMA's data quality management model, it is the process by which data elements are accumulated

Collective bargaining: A process through which a contract is negotiated that sets forth the relationship between the employees and the healthcare organization

College of American Pathologists (CAP): A medical specialty organization of board-certified pathologists that owns and holds the copyright to SNOMED CT®

College of Healthcare Information Management Executives (CHIME): A membership association serving chief information officers through professional development and advocacy

Column/field: A basic fact within a table, such as LAST_NAME, FIRST_NAME, and date of birth

Commission for the Accreditation of Freestanding Birth Centers: A group that surveys and accredits freestanding birth centers

Commission on Accreditation of Health Informatics and Information Management Education (CAHIIM): The accrediting organization for educational programs in health informatics and information management

Commission on Accreditation of Rehabilitation Facilities (CARF): A private, not-for-profit organization that develops customer-focused standards for behavioral healthcare and medical rehabilitation programs and accredits such programs on the basis of its standards

Commission on Cancer (CoC): Established by the American College of Surgeons in 1922, this entity sets standards for quality multidisciplinary cancer care. These programs are concerned with prevention, early diagnosis, pretreatment evaluation, staging, and optimal treatment, as well as rehabilitation, surveillance for recurrent disease, support services, and end-of-life care

Commission on Certification for Health Informatics and Information Management (CCHIIM): An independent body within AHIMA that establishes and enforces standards for the certification and certification maintenance of health informatics and information management professionals

Commodity: An article of trade or commerce; especially a product that is essentially the same from one vendor to another

Common-cause variation: The source of variation in a process that is inherent within the process

Common law: Unwritten law originating from court decisions where no applicable statute exists; *See* **case law; judge-made law**

Common Object Request Broker Architecture (CORBA): A component computer technology developed by a large consortium of vendors and users for handling objects over a network from various distributed platforms; the subset of standards for healthcare covered in CORBAmed

Common rule: A rule of medical ethics concerning human research and testing governed by the Institutional Review Boards

Communicable disease: A disease that can be transmitted from an infected person, animal, or inanimate reservoir to a susceptible person or host by either direct or indirect contact

Communications: The manner in which various individual computer systems are connected (for example, telephone lines, microwave, satellite)

Communications plan: A documented approach to identifying the media and schedule for sharing information with affected parties

Communication standards: *See* **transmission standards**

Communications technology: Computer networks in an information system

Communities of Practice (CoP): A web-based electronic network for communication among members of the American Health Information Management Association

Community-acquired infection: An infectious disease contracted as the result of exposure before or after a patient's period of hospitalization

Community College Consortium: A group of identified community colleges within a geographical region whose goal is to educate health information technology professionals who will be responsible for facilitating the implementation of and support for an electronic healthcare system in the United States

Community Health Accreditation Program (CHAP): A group that surveys and accredits home healthcare and hospice organizations

Community Health Dimension (CHD): One aspect of a national health information network infrastructure that acknowledges the importance of population-based health data and resources that are necessary to improve public health

Community health information network (CHIN): An integrated collection of computer and telecommunications capabilities that facilitates communications of patient, clinical, and payment information among multiple providers, payers, employers, and related healthcare entities within a community; *Also called* **community health management information system**

Community health management information system: *See* **community health information network**

Community (-based premium) rating: Method of determining healthcare insurance premium rates by geographic area (community) rather than by age, health status, or company size, which increases the size of the risk pool resulting in increased costs to younger, healthier individuals who are, in effect, subsidizing older or less healthy individuals

Comorbidity: 1. A medical condition that coexists with the primary cause for hospitalization and affects the patient's treatment and length of stay 2. Pre-existing condition that, because of its presence with a specific diagnosis, causes an increase in length of stay by at least one day in approximately 75 percent of the cases (as in complication and comorbidity [CC])

Compact disc (CD): Plastic encased disc that uses a finely focused laser beam to write and read data

Compensable factor: A characteristic used to compare the worth of jobs (for example, skill, effort, responsibility, and working conditions)

Compensation: All direct and indirect pay, including wages, mandatory benefits, and benefits such as medical insurance, life insurance, child care, elder care, retirement plans, and longevity pay

Competencies: Demonstrated skills that a worker should perform at a high level

Competent adult: An individual who has reached the age of majority and is mentally and physically competent to tend to his or her own affairs; may consent to treatment and may authorize the access or disclosure of his/her health information

Compiler: 1. A type of software that looks at an entire high-level program before translating it into machine language 2. A third-generation programming language

Complaint: In litigation, a written legal statement from a plaintiff that initiates a civil lawsuit

Complementary and alternative medicine (CAM): A group of diverse medical and healthcare systems, practices, and products that are not considered to be part of conventional medicine

Complete EHR: Under meaningful use, EHR technology that has been developed to meet, at a minimum, all applicable certification criteria adopted by the Secretary of HHS; *See also* **certified EHR**

Complete master census: A total census for a facility showing the names and locations of patients present in the hospital at a particular point in time

Completeness: An element of a legally defensible health record; the health record is not complete until all its parts are assembled and the appropriate documents are authenticated according to medical staff bylaws

Complex review: In a revenue audit contractor (RAC) review, this type of review results in an overpayment or underpayment determination based on a review of the health record associated with the claim in question

Compliance: 1. The process of establishing an organizational culture that promotes the prevention, detection, and resolution of instances of conduct that do not conform to federal, state, or private payer healthcare program requirements or the healthcare organization's ethical and business policies 2. The act of adhering to official requirements 3. Managing a coding or billing department according to the laws, regulations, and guidelines that govern it

Compliance officer: Designated individual who monitors the compliance process at a healthcare facility

Compliance plan: A process that helps an organization, such as a hospital, accomplish its goal of providing high-quality medical care and efficiently operating a business under various laws and regulations

Compliance program guidance: The information provided by the Office of the Inspector General of the Department of Health and Human Services to help healthcare organizations develop internal controls that promote adherence to applicable federal and state guidelines

Complication: 1. A medical condition that arises during an inpatient hospitalization (for example, a postoperative wound infection) 2. Condition that arises during the hospital stay that prolongs the length of stay at least one day in approximately 75 percent of the cases (as in complication and comorbidity [CC])

Complications/comorbidities (CC): Illnesses or injuries that coexist with the condition for which the patient is primarily seeking healthcare

Component alignment model (CAM): A model for strategic information systems planning that includes seven major interdependent components that should be aligned with other components in the organization

Component state associations (CSAs): Component state associations are part of the volunteer structure of AHIMA and are organized in every state, the District of Columbia, and the Commonwealth of Puerto

Rico. The purpose of each Component State Association shall be to promote the mission and purpose of AHIMA in its state

Components: Self-contained miniapplications that are an outgrowth of object-oriented computer programming and provide an easy way to expand, modernize, or customize large-scale applications because they are reusable and less prone to bugs

Comprehensive Accreditation Manual for Hospitals (CAMH): Accreditation manual published by the Joint Commission

Comprehensive Drug Abuse Prevention and Control Act of 1970: *See* **Controlled Substances Act**

Comprehensive outpatient program: In mental health or drug and alcohol treatment centers, an outpatient program for the prevention, diagnosis, and treatment of any illness, defect, or condition that prevents the individual from functioning in an optimal manner

Compressed workweek: A work schedule that permits a full-time job to be completed in less than the standard five days of eight-hour shifts

Compression algorithm: The process or program for reducing data to reduce the space needed for transmission and storage

Computer-assisted coding (CAC): The process of extracting and translating dictated and then transcribed free-text data (or dictated and then computer-generated discrete data) into ICD-9-CM and CPT evaluation and management codes for billing and coding purposes; *See also* **autocoding**

Computer-based health record: *See* **electronic health record**

Computer-based patient record: *See* **electronic health record**

Computer-based training: A type of training that is delivered partially or completely using a computer

Computer key: A number unique to a specific individual for purposes of authentication

Computer output to laser disk/enterprise report management (COLD/ERM): Technology that electronically stores documents and distributes them with fax, e-mail, web, and traditional hard-copy print processes

Computer on wheels (COWs): Term affectionately used to refer to notebook computers mounted on carts and moved with the users

Computer system security: The protection of computer hardware, software, and data from accidental or malicious access, use, modification, destruction, and/or disclosure

Computer–telephone integration (CTI): An integration of computer technology and public telephone services that allows people to access common computer functions such as database queries via telephone handsets or interactive voice technology

Computer telephony: A combination of computer and telephone technologies that allows people to use a telephone handset to access information stored in a computer system or to use computer technology to place calls within the public telephone network

Computer virus: 1. A software program that attacks computer systems with the intention of damaging or destroying files 2. Intentional computer tampering programs that may include file infectors, system or boot-record infectors, and macro viruses

Computerized internal fee schedule: The listing of the codes and associated fees maintained in the practice's computer system, along with the additional data fields necessary for completing the CMS-1500 claim form

Computerized provider order entry (CPOE): Electronic prescribing systems that allow physicians to write prescriptions and transmit them electronically. These systems usually contain error prevention software that provides the user with prompts that warn against the possibility of drug interaction, allergy, or overdose and other relevant information

CON: *See* **certificate of need**

Concept: A unique unit of knowledge or thought created by a unique combination of characteristics

Concept orientation: Concepts in a controlled medical terminology are based on meanings, not words

Concept permanence: Codes that represent the concept in a controlled medical terminology are not reused; therefore meanings do not change

Conceptual data model: The highest level of data model, representing the highest level of abstraction, independent of hardware and software

Conceptual framework of accounting: The concept that the benefits of financial data should exceed the cost of obtaining them and that the data must be understandable, relevant, reliable, and comparable

Conceptual skills: One of the three managerial skill categories that includes intellectual tasks and abilities such as planning, deciding, and problem solving

Concept Unique Identifier (CUI): A numeric identifier in RxNorm that designates the same concept, no matter the form of the name or the table where it is located; also represents an opaque identifier found in the UMLS Metathesaurus

Conclusion validity: In research, the extent to which the statistical conclusions about the relationships in the data are reasonable

Conclusive research: A type of research performed in order to come to some sort of conclusion or help in decision making; includes descriptive research and causal research

Concomitant: Accessory; taking place at the same time

Concurrent analysis: A review of the health record while the patient is still hospitalized or under treatment

Concurrent coding: A type of coding that takes place while the patient is still in the hospital and receiving care

Concurrent conditions: The physical disorders present at the same time as the primary diagnosis that alter the course of the treatment required or lengthen the expected recovery time of the primary condition

Concurrent utilization review: An evaluation of the medical necessity, quality, and cost-effectiveness of a hospital admission and ongoing patient care at or during the time that services are rendered

Conditions for Coverage: Standards applied to facilities that choose to participate in federal government reimbursement programs such as Medicare and Medicaid; *See* **Conditions of Participation**

Conditions of Participation: The administrative and operational guidelines and regulations under which facilities are allowed to take part in the Medicare and Medicaid programs; published by the Centers for Medicare and Medicaid Services, a federal agency under the Department of Health and Human Services; *Also called* **Conditions for Coverage**

Confidence interval: A healthcare statistic that is calculated from the standard error of the mean, it is an estimate of the true limits within which the true population mean lies; the range of values that may reasonably contain the true population mean

Confidential communication: As defined by HIPAA, a request that PHI be routed to an alternative location or by an alternative method

Confidentiality: A legal and ethical concept that establishes the healthcare provider's responsibility for protecting health records and other personal and private information from unauthorized use or disclosure

Configuration management: The process of keeping a record of changes made in an EHR system as it is being customized to the organization's specifications; *Also called* **change control**

Conflict management: A problem-solving technique that focuses on working with individuals to find a mutually acceptable solution

Confounding variable: In research an event or a factor that is outside a study but occurs concurrently with the study; *Also called* **extraneous variable**; **secondary variable**

Connecting For Health: A public-private collaborative designed to address the barriers to development of an interconnected health information infrastructure

Connectivity: The ability of one computer system to exchange meaningful data with another computer system

Consent: 1. A patient's acknowledgement that he or she understands a proposed intervention, including that intervention's risks, benefits, and alternatives 2. The document signed by the patient that indicates agreement that protected health information (PHI) can be disclosed

Consent directive: A process by which patients may opt in or opt out of having their data exchanged in the HIE

Consent management: Policies, procedures, and technology that enable active management and enforcement of users' consent directives to control access to their electronic health information and allow care providers to meet patient privacy requirements

Consent to treatment: Legal permission given by a patient or a patient's legal representative to a healthcare provider that allows the provider to administer care and/or treatment or to perform surgery and/or other medical procedures

Consent to use and disclose information: A written statement of permission given by a patient to a healthcare provider that allows the provider to use or disclose healthcare information for the purposes of treatment, payment, and healthcare operations

Conservatism: The concept that resources must not be overstated and liabilities not understated

Consideration: The leadership orientation of having concern for people and providing support

Consistency: The idea that all time periods must reflect the same accounting rules

Consolidated billing/bundling: A feature of the prospective payment system established by the Balanced Budget Act of 1997 for home health services provided to Medicare beneficiaries that requires the home health provider that developed the patient's plan of care to assume Medicare billing responsibility for all of the home health services the patient receives to carry out the plan

Consolidated Health Informatics (CHI): The notion of adopting existing health information interoperability standards throughout all federal agencies

Consolidated Health Informatics (CHI) initiative: The effort to achieve CHI through federal agencies spearheaded by the Office of National Coordinator for Health Information Technology

Consolidated Omnibus Budget Reconciliation Act of 1986 (COBRA): The federal law requiring every hospital that participates in Medicare and has an emergency room to treat any patient in an emergency condition or active labor, whether or not the patient is covered by Medicare and regardless of the patient's ability to pay; COBRA also requires employers to provide continuation benefits to specified workers and families who have been terminated but previously had healthcare insurance benefits

Consolidation: The process by which the ambulatory patient group classification system determines whether separate payment is appropriate when a patient is assigned multiple significant procedure groups

Constitution: A document that defines and lays out the powers of a government; considered the supreme law of that government

Constitutional law: The body of law that deals with the amount and types of power and authority that governments are given

Constructive confrontation: A method of approaching conflict in which both parties meet with an objective third party to explore perceptions and feelings

Construct validity: The ability of an instrument to measure hypothetical, nonobservable traits

Consultation: The response by one healthcare professional to another healthcare professional's request to provide recommendations and/or opinions regarding the care of a particular patient or resident

Consultation rate: The total number of hospital inpatients receiving consultations for a given period divided by the total number of discharges and deaths for the same period

Consultation report: Health record documentation that describes the findings and recommendations of consulting physicians

Consulting agencies: Companies outside the healthcare organization that provide assistance with various issues, including security awareness training

Consumer: A person who purchases and/or uses goods or services; in healthcare, a patient, client, resident, or other recipient of healthcare services

Consumer awareness campaign: The AHIMA campaign that educates the consumer about the importance of and need for a personal health record

Consumer Coalition for Health Privacy: Affiliated with the Health Privacy Project, this organization was created to educate and empower healthcare consumers on privacy issues at the various levels of government and consists of patients and consumer advocacy organizations

Consumer-directed (driven) healthcare plan (CDHP): Managed care organization characterized by influencing patients and clients to select cost-efficient healthcare through the provision of information about health benefit packages and through financial incentives

Consumer health informatics: The branch of health informatics that addresses the needs of the consumer

Consumer informatics: The field of information science concerned with the management of data and information used to support consumers by consumers (the general public) through the application of computers and computer technologies

Content: The substantive or meaningful components of a document or collection of documents

Content analysis: A method of research that provides a systematic and objective analysis of communication effectiveness, such as the analysis performed on tests

Content and records management: The management of digital and analog records using computer equipment and software. It encompasses two related organization-wide roles: content management and records management

Content validity: The extent to which an instrument's items represent the content that the instrument is intended to measure

Context: The text that illustrates a concept or the use of a designation

Context-based access control: An access control system which limits users to accessing information not only in accordance with their identity and role, but to the location and time in which they are accessing the information

Contextual: The condition of depending on the parts of a written or spoken statement that precede or follow a specified word or phrase and can influence its meaning or effect

Contingency: A plan of action to be taken when circumstances affect project performance

Contingency model of leadership: A leadership theory based on the idea that the success of task- or relationship-oriented leadership depends on leader–member relationships, task structure, and position power

Contingency plan: 1. Documentation of the process for responding to a system emergency, including the performance of backups, the line-up of critical alternative facilities to facilitate continuity of operations, and the process of recovering from a disaster 2. A recovery plan in the event of a power failure, disaster, or other emergency that limits or eliminates access to facilities and electronic protected personal health information (ePHI); *See* **business continuity plan**

Continued-stay utilization review: A periodic review conducted during a hospital stay to determine whether the patient continues to need acute care services

Continuing care retirement community: An organization established to provide housing and services, including healthcare, to people of retirement age

Continuing education: Training that enables employees to remain current with advancing knowledge in their profession

Continuing medical education (CME): Activities such as accredited sponsorship, nonaccredited sponsorship, medical teaching, and publications that advance medical care and other learning experiences, proof of which is required for a physician to maintain certification

Continuity of Care Document (CCD): The result of ASTM's Continuity of Care Record standard content being represented and mapped into the HL7's Clinical Document Architecture specifications to enable transmission of referral information between providers; also frequently adopted for personal health records

Continuity of care record (CCR): Documentation of care delivery from one healthcare experience to another

Continuous data: In healthcare statistics, data that represent measurable quantities but are not restricted to certain specified values

Continuous improvement: *See* **continuous quality improvement**

Continuous monitoring: The regular and frequent assessment of healthcare processes and their outcomes and related costs

Continuous quality improvement (CQI): 1. A management philosophy that emphasizes the importance of knowing and meeting customer expectations, reducing variation within processes, and relying on data to build knowledge for process improvement 2. A component of total quality management (TQM) that emphasizes ongoing performance assessment and improvement planning

Continuous record review: *See* **open-record review**

Continuous speech recognition: *See* **continuous speech technology**

Continuous speech technology: A computer technology that automatically translates voice patterns into written language in real time; *Also called* **continuous speech recognition**; *See* **voice recognition technology**

Continuous variables: Discrete variables measured with sufficient precision

Continuum of care: The range of healthcare services provided to patients, from routine ambulatory care to intensive acute care; the emphasis is on treating individual patients at the level of care required by their course of treatment with the assurance of communication between caregivers

Contra-account: Any account set up to adjust the historical value of a balance sheet account (for example, cumulative depreciation is a contra-account to an equipment [fixed-asset] account)

Contract: 1. A legally enforceable agreement 2. An agreement between a union and an employer that spells out details of the relationship of management and the employees

Contract coder: A coder who is hired as an independent contractor on a temporary basis to assist with coding backlog

Contracted discount rate: A type of fee-for-service reimbursement in which the third-party payer has negotiated a reduced ("discounted") fee for its covered parties; *See* **discounted fee-for-service**

Contract law: A branch of law based on common law that deals with written or oral agreements that are enforceable through the legal system

Contract service: An entity that provides certain agreed-upon services for the facility, such as transcription, coding, or copying

Contractual allowance: The difference between what is charged by the healthcare provider and what is paid by the managed care company or other payer; *Also called* contractual adjustment

Contrast material: An ingested or injected substance that enhances the appearance of anatomical structures when they undergo imaging

Control: 1. One of the four management functions in which performance is monitored in accordance with organizational policies and procedures 2. Stopping or attempting to stop postprocedural bleeding. If performing another root operation such as bypass, detachment, excisio, extraction, reposition, replacement or resection is required to stop the postprocedural bleeding, then it is not coded separately

Control chart: A run chart with lines on it called control limits that provides information to help predict the future outcome of a process with a high degree of accuracy; shows variation in key processes over time

Control group: A comparison study group whose members do not undergo the treatment under study

Controllable costs: Costs that can be influenced by a department director or manager

Controlled medical terminology: A coded vocabulary of medical concepts and expressions used in healthcare

Controlled Substances Act: The legislation that controls the use of narcotics, depressants, stimulants, and hallucinogens; *See* **Comprehensive Drug Abuse Prevention and Control Act of 1970**

Controlled vocabulary: A predefined set of terms and their meanings that may be used in structured data entry or natural language processing to represent expressions

Controlling: The monitoring and maintenance of a project's structure

Controls: 1. Subjects used for comparison who are not given a treatment under study or do not have the condition or risk factor that is the object of study 2. In disaster planning the process or plans to mitigate and reduce potential risks

Convenience sample: A type of nonrandom sampling in which researchers use any unit at hand

Convenience sampling: A sampling technique where the selection of units from the population is based on easy availability and/or accessibility

Conversion factor: A national dollar amount that Congress designates to convert relative value units to dollars; updated annually

Conversion strategy: An organization's plan for changing from a paper-based health record to an electronic health record

COO: *See* **chief operating officer**

Cookie: A piece of information passed from a web server to the user's web browser that is accessible only to the server/domain that sent it and is retrieved automatically through a program called an intelligent agent whenever the server's web page is visited; used to store passwords and ordering information and to set preferences and bookmarks

Cooperating parties for ICD-9-CM: A group of organizations (the American Health Information Management Association, the American Hospital Association, the Centers for Medicare and Medicaid Services, and the National Center for Health Statistics) that collaborates in the development and maintenance of the International Classification of Diseases, Ninth Revision, Clinical Modification (ICD-9-CM)

Coordinated care plans: Organized patient care plans that meet the standards set forth in the law for managed care plans (for example, health maintenance organizations, provider-sponsored organizations, and preferred provider organizations)

Coordination of benefits (COB): A method of integrating benefits payments from all health insurance sources to ensure that they do not exceed 100 percent of a plan member's allowable medical expenses

Coordination of benefits (COB) transaction: The electronic transmission of claims and/or payment information from a healthcare provider to a health plan for the purpose of determining relative payment responsibilities

CoP: *See* **Community of Practice**

COP: *See* **Medicare Conditions of Participation**

Copayment: Cost-sharing measure in which the policy or certificate holder pays a fixed dollar amount (flat fee) per service, supply, or procedure that is owed to the healthcare facility by the patient. The fixed amount that the policyholder pays may vary by type of service, such as $20.00 per prescription or $15.00 per physician office visit

Copy/Paste Functionality: The act of copying text within the electronic health record, copying of text from an outside document and pasting it into the EHR, and/or pasting it to a new location with the record, in which the original text is not removed from the record

CORBA: *See* **Common Object Request Broker Architecture**

Core-based statistical area (CBSA): Statistical geographic entity consisting of the county or counties associated with at least one core (urbanized area or urban cluster)

of at least 10,000 in population, plus adjacent counties having a high degree of social and economic integration with the core as measured through commuting ties with the counties containing the core. Metropolitan and micropolitan statistical areas are two components of CBSAs

Core data elements/core content: A small set of data elements with standardized definitions often considered to be the core of data collection efforts

Core measure/core measure set: Standardized performance measures developed to improve the safety and quality of healthcare (for example, core measures are used in the Joint Commission's ORYX initiative)

Coronary care unit (CCU): A facility dedicated to the care of patients who suffer from heart attacks, strokes, or other serious cardiopulmonary problems

Coroner: Typically an appointed or elected official, who may or may not be a physician, with responsibility for investigating suspicious deaths

Coroner's case: A death that appears to be suspicious and requires action from the coroner to determine the cause of death

Corporate Code of Conduct: A part of the compliance plan that expresses the organization's commitment to ethical behavior

Corporate compliance program: 1. A facility-wide program that comprises a system of policies, procedures, and guidelines that are used to ensure ethical business practices, identify potential fraudulence, and improve overall organizational performance 2. A program that became common after the Federal Sentencing Guidelines reduced fines and penalties to organizations found guilty of fraud if the organization has a prevention and detection program in place

Corporate Integrity Agreement (CIA): A compliance program imposed by the government, which involves substantial government oversight and outside expert involvement in the organization's compliance activities and is generally required as a condition of settling a fraud and abuse investigation

Corporate negligence: The failure of an organization to exercise the degree of care considered reasonable under the circumstances that resulted in an unintended injury to another party

Corporation: An organization that may have one or many owners in which profits may be held or distributed as dividends (income paid to the owners)

Correct Coding Initiative (CCI): A national initiative designed to improve the accuracy of Part B claims processed by Medicare carriers

Correction, addendum, and appending health records policy: A policy that outlines how corrections, addenda, or appendages are made in a health record

Corrective action plan (CAP): A written plan of action to be taken in response to identified issues or citations from an accrediting or licensing body

Corrective controls: Internal controls designed to fix problems that have been discovered, frequently as a result of detective controls

Correlation: The existence and degree of relationships among factors

Correlational research: A design of research that determines the existence and degree of relationships among factors

COS: *See* **clinical outcomes system**

Cost: 1. The amount of financial resources consumed in the provision of healthcare services 2. The dollar amount of a service provided by a facility

Cost accounting: The specialty branch of accounting that deals with quantifying the resources expended to provide the goods and/or services offered by the organization to its customer, client, or patients

Cost allocation: The distribution of costs

Cost–benefit analysis: A process that uses quantitative techniques to evaluate and measure the benefit of providing products or services compared to the cost of providing them

Cost centers: Groups of activities for which costs are specified together for management purposes

Cost driver: An activity that affects or causes costs

Cost inlier: A case in which the cost of treatment falls within the established cost boundaries of the assigned ambulatory patient group payment

Cost justification: A rationale developed to support competing requests for limited resources

Cost object: A product, process, department, or activity for which a healthcare organization wishes to estimate the cost

Cost of capital: The rate of return required to undertake a project

Cost-of-living adjustment (COLA): Alteration that reflects a change in the consumer price index (CPI), which measures purchasing power between time periods; the CPI is based on a market basket of goods and services that a typical consumer buys

Cost outlier: Exceptionally high costs associated with inpatient care when compared with other cases in the same diagnosis-related group

Cost outlier adjustment: Additional reimbursement for certain high-cost home care cases based on the loss-sharing ratio of costs in excess of a threshold amount for each home health resource group

Cost report: A report required from providers on an annual basis in order for the Medicare program to make a proper determination of amounts payable to providers under its provisions; analyzes the direct and indirect costs of providing care to Medicare patients

Cost-sharing: Provision of a healthcare insurance policy that requires policyholders to pay for a portion of their healthcare services; a cost-control mechanism

Council for Affordable Quality Healthcare (CAQH): A not-for-profit collaborative alliance of the nation's leading health plans and networks with a mission to improve healthcare access and quality for patients and reduce administrative burdens for healthcare providers and their office staff

Council on Accreditation (COA): A private not-for-profit organization that accredits child and family service and behavioral healthcare programs using preestablished standards and criteria

Council on Certification: An arm of AHIMA that today fulfills the role of the Board of Registration, a certification board instituted in 1933 to provide a baseline by which to measure qualified medical record librarians

Counterclaim: In a court of law, a countersuit

Countersignature: Authentication by a second provider that signifies review and evaluation of the actions and documentation, including authentication, of a first provider

Court/law enforcement referral: *See* **source of admission**

Court of Appeals: A branch of the federal court system that has the power to hear appeals on the final judgments of district courts

Court of Claims: A federal or state court in which legal actions against the government are brought

Court order: An official direction issued by a court judge and requiring or forbidding specific parties to perform specific actions

Court-ordered warrant (bench warrant): An authorization issued by a court for the attachment or arrest of a person either in the case of contempt or where an indictment has been found or to bring in a witness who does not obey a subpoena

Covered condition: In healthcare reimbursement, a health condition, illness, injury, disease, or symptom for which the healthcare insurance company will pay

Covered entity (CE): Any healthcare provider or contractor that transmits individually identifiable health information in electronic form

Covered service (expense): Specific healthcare charges that an insurer will consider for payment under the terms of a health insurance policy; *See* **benefit**

COWs: *See* **computers on wheels**

CPA: *See* **certified public accountant**

CPC: *See* **Certified Professional Coder**

CPG: *See* **Clinical practice guideline**

CPHIMS: *See* **certified professional in health information management systems**

CPOE: *See* **computerized provider order entry**

CPR charge payment method: *See* **customary, prevailing and reasonable charge payment method**

CPT: *See* **Current Procedural Terminology**

CPT Assistant: The official publication of the American Medical Association that addresses CPT coding issues

CQI: *See* **continuous quality improvement**

Creation: Making a new genital structure that does not physically take the place of a body part. Used to code sex change operations in ICD-10-PCS

Credential: A formal agreement granting an individual permission to practice in a profession, usually conferred by a national professional organization dedicated to a specific area of healthcare practice; or the accordance of permission by a healthcare organization to a licensed, independent practitioner (physician, nurse practitioner, or other professional) to practice in a specific area of specialty within that organization. Usually requires an applicant to pass an examination to obtain the credential initially and then to participate in continuing education activities to maintain the credential thereafter

Credentialing: The process of reviewing and validating the qualifications (degrees, licenses, and other credentials) of physicians and other licensed independent practitioners, for granting medical staff membership to provide patient care services

Credential verification organization (CVO): An organization that verifies healthcare professionals' background, licensing, and schooling, and tracks continuing education and other performance measures

Creditable coverage: Prior healthcare coverage that is taken into account to determine the allowable length of pre-existing condition exclusion periods (for individuals entering group health plan coverage)

Credited coverage: Reduction of waiting period for pre-existing condition based on previous creditable coverage

Credits: In accounting, or the revenue cycle, the amounts on the right side of a journal entry

CRGs: *See* **clinical risk groups**

Criminal law: A branch of law that addresses crimes that are wrongful acts against public health, safety, and welfare, usually punishable by imprisonment and/or fine

Criminal proceeding: An action instituted and conducted for the purpose of preventing the commission of a crime or for fixing the guilt of a crime already committed and punishing the offender

Crisis management plan: In disaster planning, a plan that defines the processes and controls that will be followed until the operations are fully restored

Criterion: *See* **indicator**

Critic: A role in organizational innovation in which an idea is challenged, compared to stringent criteria, and tested against reality

Critical access hospitals (CAHs): 1. Hospitals that are excluded from the outpatient prospective payment system because they are paid under a reasonable cost-based system as required under section 1834(g)

of the Social Security Act 2. Small facilities that give limited outpatient and inpatient hospital services to people in rural areas

Critical care: The care of critically ill patients in a medical emergency requiring the constant attention of the physician

Critical care services: Evaluation and management of critically ill or critically injured patients

Critical path or critical pathway: The sequence of tasks that determine the project finish date; *See* **Care Map®; clinical pathway**

Critical performance measures: A quantitative tool used to assess the importance of clinical, financial, and utilization aspects in relation to a healthcare provider's outcomes

CRM: *See* **customer relationship management; Galen Common Reference Model**

CRNA: *See* **Certified Registered Nurse Anesthetist**

Cross-claim: 1. In law, a complaint filed against a codefendant 2. A claim by one party against another party who is on the same side of the main litigation

Cross-functional: A term used to describe an entity or activity that involves more than one healthcare department, service area, or discipline

Cross-sectional study: A biomedical research study in which both the exposure and the disease outcome are determined at the same time in each subject; *See* **prevalence study**

Cross-training: The training to learn a job other than the employee's primary responsibility

Crosswalks: Lists of translating codes from one system to another

Crude birth rate: The number of live births divided by the population at risk

Crude death rate: The total number of deaths in a given population for a given period of time divided by the estimated population for the same period of time

Cryptography: 1. The art of keeping data secret through the use of mathematical or logical functions that transform intelligible data into seemingly unintelligible data and back again 2. The study of encryption and decryption techniques

CSO: *See* **chief security officer**

CT: Computed tomography

CTI: *See* **computer–telephone integration**

CTS: Carpal tunnel syndrome

CTV3: *See* **Clinical Terms, Version 3**

CUI: *See* **Concept Unique Identifier**

Cultural competence: Skilled in awareness, understanding, and acceptance of beliefs and values of the people of groups other than one's own

Current assets: Cash and other assets that typically will be converted to cash within one year

Current Dental Terminology (CDT): A medical code set of dental procedures, maintained and copyrighted by the American Dental Association (ADA), referred to as the Uniform Code on Dental Procedures and Nomenclatures until 1990

Current Procedural Terminology (CPT): A comprehensive, descriptive list of terms and associated numeric and alphanumeric codes used for reporting diagnostic and therapeutic procedures and other medical services performed by physicians; published and updated annually by the American Medical Association

Current Procedural Terminology (CPT) Category I Code: A CPT code that represents a procedure or service that is consistent with contemporary medical practice and is performed by many physicians in clinical practice in multiple locations

Current Procedural Terminology (CPT) Category II Code: A CPT code the represents services and/or test results that contribute to positive health outcomes and quality patient care

Current Procedural Terminology (CPT) Category III Code: A CPT code that represents emerging technologies for which a Category I code has yet to be established

Current ratio: The total current assets divided by total current liabilities

Curriculum: A prescribed course of study in an educational program

Custodial care: A type of care that is not directed toward a cure or restoration to a previous state of health but includes medical or nonmedical services provided to maintain a given level of health without skilled nursing care

Custodian of health records: The person designated as responsible for the operational functions of the development and maintenance of the health record and who may certify through affidavit or testimony the normal business practices used to create and maintain the record

Customary fee: The fee normally charged by physicians of the same specialty in the same geographic area

Customary, prevailing and reasonable (CPR) charge payment method: Type of retrospective fee-for-service payment method used by Medicare until 1992 to determine payment amounts for physician services, in which the third-party payer pays for fees that are customary, prevailing, and reasonable

Customer: An internal or external recipient of services, products, or information

Customer relationship management (CRM): A management system whereby organizational structure and culture and customer information and technology are aligned with business strategy so that all customer interactions can be conducted to the long-term satisfaction of the customer and to the benefit and profit of the organization

Customer service training: Training that focuses on creating a true customer orientation within the work environment

Cutover: In disaster planning, the transition process when switching from the alternative recovery site back to the original location or to a new location

CVO: *See* **credential verification organization**

CWF: Common working file

CWLA: *See* **Child Welfare League of America**

CWW: *See* **clinic without walls**

CY: *See* **calendar year**

Cybernetic systems: Systems that have standards, controls, and feedback mechanisms built in to them

Cyclical staffing: A transitional staffing solution wherein workers are brought in for specific projects or to cover in busy times

D&C: Dilation and curettage

Daily inpatient census: The number of inpatients present at census-taking time each day, plus any inpatients who were both admitted and discharged after the census-taking time the previous day

Dashboards: Reports of process measures to help leaders follow progress to assist with strategic planning; *Also called* **scorecards**

Data: The dates, numbers, images, symbols, letters, and words that represent basic facts and observations about people, processes, measurements, and conditions

Data abstracts: A defined and standardized set of data points or elements common to a patient population that can be regularly identified in the health records of the population and coded for use and analysis in a database management system

Data accessibility: Data items that are easily obtainable and legal to access with strong protections and controls built into the process

Data accuracy: The extent to which data are free of identifiable errors

Data administrator: An emerging role responsible for managing the less technical aspects of data, including data quality and security

Data analysis: The process of translating data into meaningful information

Data analyst: *See* **health data analyst**

Data audit: An organizational procedure for monitoring the quality of data by analyzing reports for anomalies, inaccuracies, and missing data

Data availability: The extent to which healthcare data are accessible whenever and wherever they are needed

Data backup plan: A plan that ensures the recovery of information that has been lost or becomes inaccessible

Data capture: The process of recording healthcare-related data in a health record system or clinical database

Data cleaning: The process of checking internal consistency and duplication as well as identifying outliers and missing data; *Also called* data cleansing; data scrubbing

Data collection: The process by which data are gathered

Data comparability: The standardization of vocabulary such that the meaning of a single term is the same each time the term is used in order to produce consistency in information derived from the data

Data comprehensiveness: All required data items are included. Ensures that the entire scope of the data is collected with intentional limitations documented

Data confidentiality: The extent to which personal health information is kept private

Data consistency: The extent to which the healthcare data are reliable and the same across applications

Data content standard: Clear guidelines for the acceptable values for specified data fields. These standards make it possible to exchange health information using electronic networks

Data conversion: The task of moving data from one data structure to another, usually at the time of a new system installation

Data cube: A collection of one or more tables of data, assembled in a fashion that allows for dynamic analysis to be conducted on the joins, intersections, and overall integration of these predefined tables stored within a data warehouse

Data currency: The extent to which data are up-to-date; a datum value is up-to-date if it is current for a specific point in time. It is outdated if it was current at some preceding time yet incorrect at a later time

Data definition: The specific meaning of a healthcare-related data element

Data definition language (DDL): A special type of software used to create the tables within a relational database, the most common of which is structured query language

Data dictionary: A descriptive list of the names, definitions, and attributes of data elements to be collected in an information system or database whose purpose is to standardize definitions and ensure consistent use

Data display: A method for presenting or viewing data

Data element: An individual fact or measurement that is the smallest unique subset of a database

Data element domain: A specification (list or range) of the valid, allowable values that can be assigned for each data element in a data set

Data Elements for Emergency Department Systems (DEEDS): A data set designed to support the uniform collection of information in hospital-based emergency departments

Data Encryption Standard (DES): A private key encryption algorithm adopted as the federal standard which uses the same private key to both encrypt and decrypt binary coded information

Data entity: a discrete form of data, such as a number or a word

Data entry: *See* **data input**

Data event: Any occurrence that generates new data or information, such as a diagnostic test

Data exchange standards: Protocols that help ensure that data transmitted from one system to another remain comparable

Data field: A predefined area within a healthcare database in which the same type of information is usually recorded

Data granularity: The level of detail at which the attributes and values of healthcare data are defined

Data input: The process of entering data into a healthcare database

Data integrity: 1. The extent to which healthcare data are complete, accurate, consistent, and timely 2. A security principle that keeps information from being modified or otherwise corrupted either maliciously or accidentally; *Also called* **data quality**

Data management: The combined practices of HIM, IT, and HI that affect how data and documentation combine to create a single business record for an organization

Data manipulation language (DML): A special type of software used to retrieve, update, and edit data in a relational database, of which the most common is structured query language

Data mart: A well-organized, user-centered, searchable database system that usually draws information from a data warehouse to meet the specific needs of users

Data miners: Those individuals who extract data from a database with the intention of quantifying and filtering the data

Data mining: The process of extracting and analyzing large volumes of data from a database for the purpose of identifying hidden and sometimes subtle relationships or patterns and using those relationships to predict behaviors

Data model: A picture or abstraction of real conditions used to describe the definitions of fields and records and their relationships in a database

Data modeling: The process of determining the users' information needs and identifying relationships among the data

Data navigator: Part of the information system development team. The person in this role would specialize in the development of the graphical user interface used to capture and navigate through the EHR and other systems

Data normalization: In a relational database, it is the process of organizing data to minimize redundancy

Data ownership: Acknowledgement by all persons involved with creating and applying data and the quality for which they are responsible

Data precision: Data values should be just large enough to support the application or process

Data quality: The reliability and effectiveness of data for its intended uses in operations, decision making, and planning; *See also* **data integrity**

Data quality indicator system: An abstracting system that records information about the patient and the care provided to the patient

Data quality management: The business processes that ensure the integrity of an organization's data during data collection, application (including aggregation), warehousing, and analysis

Data quality management model: A graphic of the data quality management domains as they relate to the characteristics of data integrity and examples of each characteristic within each domain

Data quality review: An examination of health records to determine the level of coding accuracy and to identify areas of coding problems

Data relevancy: The extent to which healthcare-related data are useful for the purposes for which they were collected

Data reliability: A measure of consistency of data items based on their reproducibility and an estimation of their error of measurement

Data repository: An open-structure database that is not dedicated to the software of any particular vendor or data supplier, in which data from diverse sources are stored so that an integrated, multidisciplinary view of the data can be achieved; *Also called* **central data repository**; when related specifically to healthcare data, a **clinical data repository**

Data resource manager: A role that ensures that the organization's information systems meet the needs of people who provide and manage patient services

Data retention: Each facility must decide how long patient-specific data will be retained. This decision must be made based on the needs of the organization, regulations, and laws

Data retrieval: The process of obtaining data from a healthcare database

Data security: The process of keeping data, both in transit and at rest, safe from unauthorized access, alteration, or destruction

Data set: A list of recommended data elements with uniform definitions that are relevant for a particular use

Data silos: Separate repositories of data that do not communicate with each other

Data standard: The agreed-upon specifications for the values acceptable for specific data fields; *See also* **data content standard**

Data stewardship: The responsibilities and accountabilities associated with managing, collecting, viewing, storing, sharing, disclosing, or otherwise making use of personal health information

Data storage: The physical location and maintenance of data

Data structure: The form in which data are stored, as in a file, a database, a data repository, and so on

Data timeliness: Concept of data quality that involves whether the data is up-to-date and available within a useful time frame. Timeliness is determined by how the data are being used and their context

Data translator: The liaison between the patient and his health data

Data type: A technical category of data (text, numbers, currency, date, memo, and link data) that a field in a database can contain

Data validity: The extent to which data have been verified to be accurate

Data warehouse: A database that makes it possible to access data from multiple databases and combine the results into a single query and reporting interface; *See* **clinical data warehouse**; **clinical repository**

Data warehouse management system (DWMS): A type of software that manages a data warehouse

Data warehousing: The acquisition of all the business data and information from potentially multiple, cross-platform sources, such as legacy databases, departmental databases, and online transaction-based databases, and then the warehouse storage of all the data in one consistent format used to analyze data for decision-making purposes

Database: An organized collection of data, text, references, or pictures in a standardized format, typically stored in a computer system for multiple applications

Database administrator: The individual responsible for the technical aspects of designing and managing databases

Data-based DSS: Decision support system that focuses on providing access to the various data sources within the organization through one system

Database life cycle (DBLC): A system consisting of several phases that represent the useful life of a database, including initial study, design, implementation, testing and evaluation, operation, and maintenance and evaluation

Database management: The process of controlling access to the information in a database that uses passwords or other access control techniques

Database management system (DBMS): Computer software that enables the user to create, modify, delete, and view the data in a database

Database model: A description of the structure to be used to organize data in a healthcare-related database such as an electronic health record

Date of birth: The year, month, and day when an individual was born

Date of encounter (outpatient and physician services): The year, month, and day of an encounter, visit, or other healthcare encounter

Date of procedure (inpatient): The year, month, and day of each significant procedure

Date of service (DOS): The date a test, procedure, and/or service was rendered

Day on leave of absence: A day occurring after the admission and prior to the discharge of a hospital inpatient when the patient is not present at the census-taking hour because he or she is on leave of absence from the healthcare facility

Day outlier: An inpatient hospital stay that is exceptionally long when compared with other cases in the same diagnosis-related group

Days in accounts receivable: The ending accounts receivable balance divided by an average day's revenues

Days of stay: *See* **length of stay**

DBLC: *See* **database life cycle**

DBMS: *See* **database management system**

DDL: *See* **data definition language**

Dead on arrival (DOA): The condition of a patient who arrives at a healthcare facility with no signs of life and who was pronounced dead by a physician

Death certificate: Paperwork that must be completed when someone dies, as directed by state law; generally filled out by the funeral director or other person responsible for internment or cremation of remains and signed by the physician, who provides the cause of death

Death rate: The proportion of inpatient hospitalizations that end in death

Debit: The amount on the left side of an account entry that represents an increase in an expense or liability account or a decrease in a revenue or asset account

Debt: Incurred when money is borrowed and must eventually be paid

Debt financing: The process of borrowing money at a cost in the form of interest

Debt ratio: The total liabilities divided by the total assets

Debt service: The current obligations of an organization to repay loans

Decentralization: The shift of decision-making authority and responsibility to lower levels of the organization

Decile: The tenth equal part of a distribution

Decimal: Numbered or proceeding by tens; based on the number 10; expressed in or utilizing a decimal system, especially with a decimal point

Decision support system (DSS): A computer-based system that gathers data from a variety of sources and assists in providing structure to the data by using various analytical models and visual tools in order to facilitate and improve the ultimate outcome in decision-making tasks associated with nonroutine and nonrepetitive problems

Decision tree: A structured data-mining technique based on a set of rules useful for predicting and classifying information and making decisions

Decommissioned: Obsolete information system or data set

Deductible: The amount of cost, usually annual, that the policyholder must incur (and pay) before the insurance plan will assume liability for remaining covered expenses

Deductive reasoning: The process of developing conclusions based on generalizations

DEEDS: *See* **Data Elements for Emergency Department Systems**

Deemed status: An official designation indicating that a healthcare facility is in compliance with the Medicare Conditions of Participation; to qualify for deemed status, facilities must be accredited by the Joint Commission or AOA

Default: 1. The status to which a computer application reverts in the absence of alternative instructions 2. Pertains to an attribute, value, or option that is assumed when none is explicitly specified

Default judgment: A court ruling against a defendant in a lawsuit who fails to answer a summons for a court appearance

Defendant: In civil cases, an individual or entity against whom a civil complaint has been filed; in criminal cases, an individual who has been accused of a crime

Deficiency analysis: An audit process designed to ensure that all services billed have been documented in the health record

Deficiency slip: A device for tracking information (for example, reports) missing from a paper-based health record

Deficiency systems: Paper- or computer-based processes designed to track and report elements of documentation missing from the health records of discharged patients

Degaussing: The process of removing or rearranging the magnetic field of a disk in order to render the data unrecoverable

Deidentification: The process in which users of secondary data will need to remove identifying data so that data can be used without violating the patient's privacy

De-identified information: Health information from which all names and other identifying descriptors have been removed to protect the privacy of the patients, family members, and healthcare providers who were involved in the case

De-identify: 1. The act of removing from a health record or data set any information that could be used to identify the individual to whom the data apply in order to protect his or her confidentiality 2. To remove the names of the principal investigator (PI), co-investigators, and affiliated organizations to allow reviewers to maintain objectivity

Delegation: The process by which managers distribute work to others along with the authority to make decisions and take action

Delegation of authority: The assignment of authority or responsibility

Delete: 1. To eliminate by blotting out, cutting out, or erasing 2. To remove or eliminate, as to erase data from a field or to eliminate a record from a file; a method of erasing data

Delinquent health record: An incomplete record not finished or made complete within the time frame determined by the medical staff of the facility

Deliverable: A tangible output produced by the completion of project tasks

Delivery: The process of delivering a live-born infant or dead fetus (and placenta) by manual, instrumental, or surgical means

Delivery room: A special operating room for obstetric delivery and infant resuscitation

Delivery system: An organized method of providing healthcare services to a large number of individuals in a geopolitical region or a contractually defined population

Demand bill: A bill generated and issued to the patient at the time of service or any other time outside the normal accounting cycle

Demographic data: *See* **demographic information**

Demographic information: Information used to identify an individual, such as name, address, gender, age, and other information linked to a specific person

Denial: When a bill has been returned unpaid for any of several reasons (for example, sending the bill to the wrong insurance company, patient not having current coverage, inaccurate coding, lack of medical necessity, and so on)

Denominator: The part of a fraction below the line signifying division that functions as the divisor of the numerator and, in fractions with 1 as the numerator, indicates into how many parts the unit is divided

Dental codes: Codes used for billing for dental procedures, classified in the Current Procedural Terminology (CPT)

Dental informatics: A field of information science concerned with the management of data and information used to support the practice and delivery of dental healthcare through the application of computers and computer technologies

Department of a provider: A facility, organization, or physician's office that is either created or acquired by a main provider for the purpose of furnishing healthcare services under the name, ownership, and financial and administrative control of the main provider, in accordance with the provisions of the ambulatory payment classification final rule

Department of Health and Human Services (HHS): The cabinet-level federal agency that oversees all the health- and human-services–related activities of the federal government and administers federal regulations

Department of Health and Human Services Office for Civil Rights (OCR): Agency within the Department of Health and Human Services responsible for civil rights and health privacy rights law enforcement

Dependency: The relationship between two tasks in a project plan

Dependent: An insured's spouse and unmarried children, claimed on income tax. The maximum age of dependent children varies by policy. A common ceiling is 19 years of age, with continuation to age 26 provided the child is a full-time student at an accredited school, primarily dependent upon the covered employee for support and maintenance, and is unmarried. Some healthcare insurance policies also allow same-sex domestic partners to be listed as dependents

Dependent variable: A measurable variable in a research study that depends on an independent variable

Deposition: A method of gathering information to be used in a litigation process

Depreciation: The allocation of the dollar cost of a capital asset over its expected life

Derived attribute: An attribute whose value is based on the value of other attributes (for example, current date minus date of birth yields the derived attribute age)

DES: *See* **Data Encryption Standard**

Description: In a controlled medical vocabulary, a description is the combination of a concept and a term

Descriptive research: A type of research that determines and reports the current status of topics and subjects

Descriptive statistics: A set of statistical techniques used to describe data such as means, frequency distributions, and standard deviations; statistical information that describes the characteristics of a specific group or a population

Descriptive text: One component of the DSM, text that describes mental disorders under the following headings: Diagnostic Features; Subtypes and/or Specifiers; Recording Procedures; Associated Features and Disorders; Specific Culture, Age, and Gender Features; Prevalence, Course, Familial Pattern, and Differential Diagnosis

Descriptor: Wording that represents the official definition of an item or service that can be billed using a particular code

Design phase: The second phase of the systems development life cycle during which all options in selecting a new information system are considered

Designated record set: A group of records maintained by or for a covered entity that may include patient medical and billing records; the enrollment, payment, claims adjudication, and cases or medical management record systems maintained by or for a health plan; or information used, in whole or in part, to make patient care–related decisions

Designated standards maintenance organizations (DSMO): A category of organization established by the Health Insurance Portability and Accountability Act to maintain the electronic transaction standards mandated by HIPAA

Destruction of records: The act of breaking down the components of a health record into pieces that can no longer be recognized as parts of the original record

DET: Detailed

Det Norske Veritas (DNV): An independent international organization that began offering hospital accreditation services in the United States in 2008

Detachment: Cutting off all or part of the upper or lower extremities. Used exclusively to code amputation procedures

Detective controls: Controls that are put in place to find errors that may have been made during a process; for example, routine coding quality audits and registration audits

Developing stage: In performance management, the stage during which opportunities for improving work processes or employee skills are identified

Development: The process of growing or progressing in one's level of skill, knowledge, or ability

Developmental disability: A mental or physical limitation affecting major life activities, arising before adulthood, and usually lasting throughout life

Device driver: A specific type of software that is made to interact with hardware devices, such as the printer driver that ensures that the computer directs printing instructions appropriate to the type of printer to which it is connected

DG: *See* **documentation guideline**

Diagnosis: A word or phrase used by a physician to identify a disease from which an individual patient suffers or a condition for which the patient needs, seeks, or receives medical care

Diagnosis-related groups (DRGs): A unit of case-mix classification adopted by the federal government and some other payers as a prospective payment mechanism for hospital inpatients in which diseases are placed into groups because related diseases and treatments tend to consume similar amounts of healthcare resources and incur similar amounts of cost; in the Medicare and Medicaid programs, one of more than 500 diagnostic classifications in which cases demonstrate similar resource consumption and length-of-stay patterns. Under the prospective payment system (PPS), hospitals are paid a set fee for treating patients in a single DRG category, regardless of the actual cost of care for the individual

Diagnostic and Statistical Manual of Mental Disorders, Fourth Revision (DSM-IV): A nomenclature developed by the American Psychiatric Association to standardize the diagnostic process for patients with psychiatric disorders, which includes codes that correspond to ICD-9-CM codes; most recent version is fourth edition (text revision), or DSM-IV-TR, published in 2000

Diagnostic and Statistical Manual of Mental Disorders, Fourth Revision, Text Revision **(DSM-IV-TR):** The 2004 text revision of the Diagnostic and Statistical Manual of Mental Disorders, Fourth Revision, with updated clinical terms, but very few coding changes

Diagnostic codes: Numeric or alphanumeric characters used to classify and report diseases, conditions, and injuries

Diagnostic criteria: For each mental disorder listed in the DSM-IV, a set of extensive diagnostic criteria are provided that indicate what symptoms must be present as well as those symptoms that must not be present in order for a patient to meet the qualifications for a particular mental diagnosis

Diagnostic image data: Bitmapped images used for medical or diagnostic purposes (for example, chest x-rays or computed tomography scans)

Diagnostic mammography: Breast imaging, either unilateral or bilateral, done to provide information on a patient with a suspected breast condition

Diagnostic services: All diagnostic services of any type, including history, physical examination, laboratory, x-ray or radiography, and others that are performed or ordered pertinent to the patient's reasons for the encounter

Dichotomous data: *See* **nominal level data**

DICOM: *See* **Digital Imaging and Communication in Medicine**

Dictation system: Used by physicians and transcription staff to dictate various medical reports such as the operative report, history and physical, and the discharge summary

Differentiation: The degree to which a tumor resembles the normal tissue from which it arose

Diffusion S curve: Curve that shows that each of the adopter categories engages innovation at a different time and a different acceptance rate

Digital: 1. A data transmission type based on data that have been binary encoded 2. A term that refers to the data or information represented in an encoded, computer-readable format

Digital certificate: An electronic document that establishes a person's online identity

Digital dictation: A process in which vocal sounds are converted to bits and stored on computer for random access

Digital images: Data provided in a computer-readable format

Digital Imaging and Communication in Medicine (DICOM): A standard that promotes a digital image communications format and picture archive and communications systems for use with digital images

Digital signature: An electronic signature that binds a message to a particular individual and can be used by the receiver to authenticate the identity of the sender

Digital signature management technology: The practice of validating the identity of an individual sending data through the use of an electronic signature

Dilation: Expanding an orifice or the lumen of a tubular body part. Coded when the objective of the procedure is to enlarge the diameter of a tubular body part or orifice

Direct costs: Resources expended that can be identified as pertaining to specific goods and/or services (for example, medications pertain to specific patients)

Direct laryngoscopy: The procedure that allows the larynx to be viewed through an endoscope

Direct medical education costs: An add-on to the ambulatory payment classification amount to compensate for costs associated with outpatient direct medical education of interns and residents

Direct method of cost allocation: Distributes the cost of overhead departments solely to the revenue-producing areas

Direct observation: A method in which the researchers conduct the observation themselves, spending time in the environment they are observing and recording observations

Direct obstetric death: The death of a woman resulting from obstetric complications of the pregnancy state, labor, or puerperium; from interventions, omissions, or treatment; or from a chain of events resulting from any of the events listed

Direct relationship: *See* **positive relationship**

Disability: A physical or mental condition that either temporarily or permanently renders a person unable to do the work for which he or she is qualified and educated

Disaster planning: A plan for protecting electronic protected health information (ePHI) in the event of a disaster that limits or eliminates access to facilities and ePHI

Disaster recovery coordinator: The individual authorized and responsible for implementing and coordinating IS disaster recovery operations

Disaster recovery plan (DRP): The document that defines the resources, actions, tasks, and data required to manage the businesses recovery process in the event of a business interruption

Discharge: The point at which an individual's active involvement with an organization or program ends, and the organization or program no longer maintains active responsibility for the care of the individual. In ambulatory or office-based settings, where episodes of care occur even though the organization continues to maintain active responsibility for the care of the individuals, discharge is the point at which an encounter or episode of care (that is, an office or clinic visit for the purpose of diagnostic evaluation or testing, procedures, treatment, therapy, or management) ends

Discharge abstract system: A data repository (usually electronic) used for collecting information on demographics, clinical conditions, and services in which data are condensed from hospital health records into coded data for the purpose of producing summary statistics about discharged patients

Discharge analysis: An analysis of the health record at or following discharge

Discharge and readmit (home health): A situation in which a home health provider receives a prorated partial episode payment for the original episode when a beneficiary is discharged and readmitted to the same agency within the same 60-day period

Discharge date (inpatient): The year, month, and day that an inpatient was formally released from the hospital and room, board, and continuous nursing services were terminated

Discharge days: *See* **length of stay; total length of stay**

Discharge diagnosis: Any one of the diagnoses recorded after all the data accumulated during the course of a patient's hospitalization or other circumscribed episode of medical care have been studied

Discharge diagnosis list: A complete set of discharge diagnoses applicable to a single patient episode, such as an inpatient hospitalization

Discharge planning: The process of coordinating the activities related to the release of a patient when inpatient hospital care is no longer needed

Discharge status: The disposition of the patient at discharge (that is, left against medical advice, discharged to home, transferred to skilled nursing facility, or died)

Discharge summary: A summary of the resident's stay at a healthcare facility that is used along with the postdischarge plan of care to provide continuity of care upon discharge from the facility

Discharge transfer: The transfer of an inpatient to another healthcare institution at the time of discharge

Discharge utilization review: A process for assessing a patient's readiness to leave the hospital

Discharged, no final bill (DNFB) report: A report that includes all patients who have been discharged from the facility but for whom, for one reason or another, the billing process is not complete

Disciplinary action: Action taken to improve unsatisfactory work performance or behavior on the job

Discipline: A field of study characterized by a knowledge base and perspective that is different from other fields of study

Disclosure: The act of making information known; in the health information management context, the release of confidential health information about an identifiable person to another person or entity

Discounted fee for service: Type of fee-for-service reimbursement in which the third-party payer has negotiated a reduced fee for its covered insureds; *See also* **contracted discount rate**

Discounting: 1. The application of lower rates of payment to multiple surgical procedures performed during the same operative session under the outpatient prospective payment system; the application of adjusted rates of payment by preferred provider organizations 2. Reducing the payment in the hospital outpatient prospective payment system (HOPPS) (payment status indicator = T). In the CMS's discounting schedule, Medicare will pay 100 percent of the Medicare allowance for the principal procedure (exclusive of deductible and copayment) and 50 percent (50 percent discount) of the Medicare allowance for each additional procedure. For example, if two CT scans (APC group 0349) are performed in the same visit, the first is reimbursed at the full APC group rate, the second at 50 percent of the APC group rate

Discoverability: Limitations on the ability of parties to discover pretrial information held by another

Discovery: *See* **discovery process**

Discovery process: The pretrial stage in the litigation process during which both parties to a suit use various strategies to identify information about the case, the primary focus of which is to determine the strength of the opposing party's case

Discovery request: Type of request that may be used to obtain information (not limited to record requests), including deposition, testimony to authenticate records, interrogatories, production of documents, physical or mental examination of a party, requests for admission, subpoenas, and court orders

Discrete data: Data that represent separate and distinct values or observations; that is, data that contain only finite numbers and have only specified values

Discrete variable: A dichotomous or nominal variable whose values are placed into categories

Discrimination: The act of treating one entity differently from another

Discus monitoring form: *See* **Antipsychotic Dyskinesia Identification System**

Disease index: A list of diseases and conditions of patients sequenced according to the code numbers of the classification system in use

Disease management (DM): Emphasizes the provider-patient relationship in the development and execution of the plan of care, prevention strategies using evidence-based guidelines to limit complications and exacerbations, and evaluation based on outcomes that support improved overall health

Disease registry: A centralized collection of data used to improve the quality of care and measure the effectiveness of a particular aspect of healthcare delivery

Disenrollment: A process of termination of coverage of a plan member

Disk mirroring: A storage technique which mirrors data from a primary drive to a secondary in the event of a drive failure

Disposition: For outpatients, the healthcare practitioner's description of the patient's status at discharge (no follow-up planned; follow-up planned or scheduled; referred elsewhere; expired); for inpatients, a core health data element that identifies the circumstances under which the patient left the hospital (discharged alive; discharged to home or self-care; discharged and transferred to another short-term general hospital for inpatient care; discharged and transferred to a skilled nursing facility; discharged and transferred to an intermediate care facility; discharged and transferred to another type of institution for inpatient care or referred for outpatient services to another institution; discharged and transferred to home under care of organized home health services organization; discharged and transferred to home under care of a home intravenous therapy provider; left against medical advice or discontinued care; expired; status not stated)

Disproportionate share hospital (DSH): Healthcare organizations that meet governmental criteria for percentages of indigent patients. Hospital with an unequally (disproportionately) large share of low-income patients. Federal payments to these hospitals are increased to adjust for the financial burden

Distance learning: A learning delivery mode in which the instructor, the classroom, and the students are not all present in the same location and at the same time

Distribution-free technique: *See* **nonparametric technique**

District court: The lowest tier in the federal court system, which hears cases involving felonies and misdemeanors that fall under federal statute and suits in which a citizen of one state sues a citizen of another state

Diversity: Any perceived difference among people, such as age, functional specialty, profession, sexual orientation, geographic origin, lifestyle, or tenure with the organization or position

Diversity jurisdiction: Refers to district court cases that involve suits where a citizen of one state sues a citizen of another state and the amount in dispute exceeds $75,000

Diversity training: A type of training that facilitates an environment that fosters tolerance and appreciation of individual differences within the organization's workforce and strives to create a more harmonious working environment

Divestiture: The result of a parent company selling a portion of the company to an outside party for cash or other assets

Dividends: The portion of an organization's profit that is distributed to its investors

Division: Cutting into a body part without draining fluids and/or gases from the body part in order to separate or transect the body part

DM: *See* **disease management**

DME: *See* **durable medical equipment**

DMERC: *See* **durable medical equipment regional carrier**

DML: *See* **data manipulation language**

DNFB report: *See* **discharged, no final bill report**

DNR: *See* **do not resuscitate**

DNV: *See* **Det Norske Veritas**

DOA: *See* **dead on arrival**

Document: Any analog or digital, formatted, and preserved "container" of data or information

Document control number (DCN): A term used to refer to the number assigned to a claim when received for processing, facilitating ease of search on the part of the CMS

Document image data: Bitmapped images based on data created and/or stored on analog paper or photographic film

Document imaging: The practice of electronically scanning written or printed paper documents into an optical or electronic system for later retrieval of the document or parts of the document if parts have been indexed

Document integrity (digital): The extent to which it can be assured that an electronic document has not been modified, altered, or deleted without proper attribution and version control; the characteristic, attribute, or extent to which an electronic document is considered to have authenticity

Document management technology: Technology that organizes, assembles, secures, and shares documents, and includes such functions as document version control, check-in and check-out control, document access control, and text and word searches

Document review: An in-depth study performed by accreditation surveyors of an organization's policies and procedures, administrative records, human resources records, performance improvement documentation, and other similar documents, as well as a review of closed patient records

Documentation: The recording of pertinent healthcare findings, interventions, and responses to treatment as a business record and form of communication among caregivers

Documentation Event Audit: A function that allows the retrospective reconstruction of documentation events, including the author, the date, the time, and the "before and after" state of the documentation

Documentation guideline (DG): A statement that indicates what health information must be recorded to substantiate use of a particular CPT code

Documentation integrity (healthcare): The characteristic or extent to which healthcare documentation adequately and accurately reflects the condition of the patient, decision-making processes of the clinician, and healthcare services that were rendered; may also refer to the extent to which healthcare documentation is protected from unauthorized use or disclosure (the maintenance of privacy and security of the documentation)

Documentation paradigm: A disease-specific format developed by the individual provider for the purpose of establishing standard clinical documentation forms

Dollars billed: The amount of money billed for services rendered

Dollars in accounts receivable: The amount of money owed a healthcare facility when claims are pending

Dollars received: Payments agreed upon through diagnosis-related group selection, contractual agreements, or other payer payment methods

Domain: A sphere or field of activity and influence

Do not resuscitate (DNR): An order written by the treating physician stating that in the event the patient suffers cardiac or pulmonary arrest, cardiopulmonary resuscitation should not be attempted

DOS: *See* **date of service**

Dose form: The form in which a drug is administered to a patient, as opposed to the form in which the manufacturer had supplied it

Double-blind study: A type of clinical trial conducted with strict procedures for randomization in which neither researcher nor subject knows whether the subject is in the control group or the experimental group

Double distribution: A budgeting concept in which overhead costs are allocated twice, taking into consideration that some overhead departments provide services to each other

Double-entry accounting: A generally accepted method for recording accounting transactions in which debits are posted in the column on the left and credits are posted in the column on the right

Downcoding: A term used to describe the process by which third-party payers or other reviews change a code on a claim to a less complex or lower-cost procedure than was originally reported

Downsizing: A reengineering strategy to reduce the cost of labor and streamline the organization by laying off portions of the workforce

Downtime procedure policy: A policy that focuses on sustaining business function during short interruptions that do not exceed the threshold that would be classified as disasters; *Also called* **contingency plan**

DPOA: *See* **durable power of attorney**

DPOA HCD: *See* **durable power of attorney for healthcare decisions**

Drainage: Taking or letting out fluids and/or gases from a body part

DRG: *See* **diagnosis-related group**

DRG creep: An increase in a case-mix index that occurs through the coding of higher-paying principal diagnoses and of more complications and comorbidities, even though the actual severity level of the patient population did not change

DRG grouper: A computer program that assigns inpatient cases to diagnosis-related groups and determines the Medicare reimbursement rate

Drivers and passengers: Exploding charges wherein the driver is the item that explodes into other items and appears on the bill

Drop-down menu: A list of options that appear below an item when clicked which a user selects to complete the computer entry; *See also* **pick list**

DRP: *See* **disaster recovery plan**

Drug components: The elements that together constitute a clinical drug

Drug Listing Act of 1972: This act amended the Federal Food, Drug, and Cosmetic Act so that drug establishments that are engaged in the manufacturing, preparation, propagation, compounding, or processing of a drug are required to register their establishments and list all of their commercially marketed drug products with the Food and Drug Administration (FDA)

DSH: *See* **disproportionate share hospital**

DSM-IV: *See* **Diagnostic and Statistical Manual of Mental Disorders, Fourth Revision**

DSM-IV-TR: *See* ***Diagnostic and Statistical Manual of Mental Disorders, Fourth Revision, Text Revision***

DSS: *See* **decision support system**

Dual core (vendor strategy): A vendor strategy in which one vendor primarily supplies the financial and administrative applications and another vendor primarily supplies the clinical applications

Dual eligible: An individual covered by both Medicare and Medicaid

Dual option: The offering of health maintenance organization coverage as well as indemnity insurance by the same carrier

Due diligence: The actions associated with making a good decision, including investigation of legal, technical, human, and financial predictions and ramifications of proposed endeavors with another party

Due process: The right of individuals to fair treatment under the law

Due process of law: The guarantee provided under the Constitution and the Bill of Rights that laws will be reasonable and not arbitrary and allows for challenges to a law's content and substance

Dumping: The illegal practice of transferring uninsured and indigent patients who need emergency services from one hospital to another (usually public) hospital solely to avoid the cost of providing uncompensated services. EMTALA, passed in 1986 and implemented in 1990, contains provisions intended to curtail this practice

Duplex scan: An ultrasonic scanning procedure that displays both two-dimensional structure and motion with time; utilizes Doppler ultrasonic signal documentation with spectral analysis and/or color flow velocity mapping or imaging

Duplicate billing: The practice of submitting more than one claim for the same item or service

Duplicate medical record number: The situation in which a single patient is associated with more than one medical record number

Durable medical equipment (DME): Medical equipment designed for long-term use in the home, including eyeglasses, hearing aids, surgical appliances and supplies, orthotics and prostheses, and bulk and cylinder oxygen; *Also called* **home medical equipment (HME)**

Durable medical equipment regional carrier (DMERC): A fiscal intermediary designated to process claims for durable medical equipment

Durable power of attorney (DPOA): A power of attorney that remains in effect even after the principal is incapacitated; some are drafted so that they only take effect when the principal becomes incapacitated

Durable power of attorney for healthcare decisions (DPOA-HCD): A legal instrument through which a principal appoints an agent to make healthcare decisions on the principal's behalf in the event the principal becomes incapacitated

Duration: The amount of time, usually measured in days, for a task to be completed

Duration of inpatient hospitalization: *See* **length of stay**

Duty: Obligation

Duty to warn: The legal obligation of a health professional to disclose information to warn an intended victim when a patient threatens to harm an individually identifiable victim and the psychiatrist or mental health provider believes that the patient is likely to harm the individual

DWMS: *See* **data warehouse management system**

DX: *See* **diagnosis**

Early adopters: Accounts for about 13.5 percent of the organization. The individuals in this group have a high degree of opinion leadership, and they are more localized than cosmopolitan and often look to the innovators for advice and information; these are the leaders and respected role models in the organization, and their adoption of an idea or practice does much to initiate change

Early fetal death: The death of a product of human conception that is fewer than 20 weeks of gestation and 500 grams or less in weight before its complete expulsion or extraction from the mother

Early majority: Compromises about 34 percent of the organization; although usually not leaders, the individuals in this group represent the backbone of the organization, are deliberate in thinking and acceptance of an idea, and serve as a natural bridge between early and late adopters

Earnings report: *See* **statement of revenue and expenses**

E code (external cause of injury code): A supplementary ICD-9-CM classification used to identify the external causes of injuries, poisonings, and adverse effects of pharmaceuticals

e-commerce: The use of the Internet and its derived technologies to integrate all aspects of business-to-business and business-to-consumer activities, processes, and communications

ECRI: An independent nonprofit health services research agency established to promote safety, quality, and cost-effectiveness in healthcare to benefit patient care through research, publishing, education, and consultation; formerly known as the Emergency Care Research Institute

ECRM: *See* **enterprise content and record management**

ECM: *See* **enterprisewide content management**

EDI: *See* **electronic data interchange**

e-Discovery: Refers to Amendments to Federal Rules of Civil Procedure and Uniform Rules Relating to Discovery of Electronically Stored Information; wherein audit trails, the source code of the program, metadata, and any other electronic information that is not typically considered the legal health record is subject to motion for compulsory discovery

Edit: A condition that must be satisfied before a computer system can accept data

Editor: Logic (algorithms) within computer software that evaluates data. Medicare's Standard Claims Processing System (or PSC Supplemental Edit Software) and its Outpatient Code Editor (OCE) contain editors that select certain claims, evaluate, or compare information on the selected claims or other accessible source, and depending on the evaluation, take actions on the claims, such as pay in full, pay in part, or suspend for manual review; *See* **code editor**

EDMS: *See* **electronic document management systems**

Educational level: The highest level, in years, within each major (primary, secondary, baccalaureate, postbaccalaureate) educational system, regardless of any certifications achieved

EEG: Electroencephalogram

Effectiveness: The degree to which stated outcomes are attained

Efficacy: The degree to which a minimum of resources is used to obtain outcomes

Efficiency: In the language of the Joint Commission, the ratio of the outcomes for a patient to the resources consumed in delivering the care

Effort: The mental and physical exertion required to perform job-related tasks

e-forms technology: *See* **automated forms processing technology**

e-health initiative: A private organization which involves many groups working on the improvement of health information technology and health information exchange

e-HIM: The application of technology to managing health information

EHR: *See* **electronic health record**

EHR collaborative: A group of healthcare professional and trade associations formed to support Health Level 7 (HL7), a healthcare standards development organization, in the development of a functional model for electronic health record systems

EHR module: Any service, component, or combination thereof that can meet the requirements of at least one certification criterion adopted by the Secretary

EHR-S: *See* **EHR system**

EHR system (EHR-S): A system that ensures the longitudinal collection of electronic health information for and about persons; enables immediate electronic access to person- and population-level information by authorized users; provides knowledge and decision support that enhance the quality, safety, and efficiency of patient care; and supports efficient processes for healthcare delivery

Eighty-five/fifteen (85/15) rule: The total quality management assumption that 85 percent of the problems that occur are related to faults in the system rather than to worker performance

EIN: *See* **employer identification number**

EIS: *See* **executive information system**

e-learning: The use of the Internet and its derived technologies to deliver training and education

Elective admission: The formal acceptance by a healthcare organization of a patient whose condition permits adequate time to schedule the availability of a suitable accommodation

Elective surgery: A classification of surgery that does not have to be performed immediately to prevent death or serious disability

Electrodesiccation: The destruction of tissue by way of a small needle heated by passing electricity through it

Electronic data interchange (EDI): A standard transmission format using strings of data for business information communicated among the computer systems of independent organizations

Electronic document management system (EDMS): A storage solution based on digital scanning technology in which source documents are scanned to create digital images of the documents that can be stored electronically on optical disks; *See* **document management technology**

Electronic health record (EHR): An electronic record of health-related information on an individual that conforms to nationally recognized interoperability standards and that can be created, managed, and consulted by authorized clinicians and staff across more than one healthcare organization

Electronic health record system (EHR-S): A system that ensures the longitudinal collection of electronic health information for and about persons; enables immediate electronic access to person- and population-level information by authorized users; provides knowledge and decision support that enhances the quality, safety, and efficiency of patient care; and supports efficient processes for healthcare delivery

Electronic medical record (EMR): An electronic record of health-related information on an individual that can be created, gathered, managed, and consulted by authorized clinicians and staff within a single healthcare organization

Electronic medication administration record (EMAR): A system designed to prevent medication errors by checking a patient's medication information against his or her bar-coded wristband

Electronic Performance Support System (EPSS): Sets of computerized tools and displays that automate training, documentation, and phone support; that integrate this automation into applications; and that provide support that is faster, cheaper, and more effective than traditional methods

Electronic prescribing (e-Rx): When a prescription is written from the personal digital assistant and an electronic fax or an actual electronic data interchange transaction is generated that transmits the prescription directly to the retail pharmacy's information system

Electronic Protected Health Information (ePHI): Under HIPAA, all individually identifiable information that is created or received electronically by a healthcare provider or any other entity subject to HIPAA requirements

Electronic record management (ERM): Systems that capture data from print files and other report-formatted digital documents, such as e-mail, e-fax, instant messages, web pages, digital dictation, and speech recognition and stores them for subsequent viewing; *Also called* computer output to laser disk (COLD) technology

Electronic remittance advice (ERA): A classification of payment information from third-party payers that is communicated electronically

Electronic signature: A generic, technology-neutral term for the various ways that an electronic record can be signed, such as a digitized image of a signature, a name typed at the end of an e-mail message by the sender, a biometric identifier, a secret code or PIN, or a digital signature

Electronic signature authentication (ESA): A system that requires the author of a document to sign onto a patient record using a user ID and password, reviews the document to be signed, and indicates approval

Electronically stored information (ESI): Data or documents, including e-mail and electronic health records, that are stored electronically rather than physically

Elements of negligence: Four basic elements must be proven in a malpractice case: failure to use due care, breach of duty, damages, and causation

Eligible hospitals—Medicare Advantage (MA): Under the EHR Incentive Program (Meaningful Use) Final Rule, hospitals which are eligible to receive incentive payments are the same as FFS EHR program

Eligible hospitals—Medicare Fee For Service (FFS): Under the EHR Incentive Program (Meaningful Use) Final Rule, hospitals which are eligible to receive incentive payments include acute care hospitals and critical access hospitals (CAH)

Eligible hospitals—Medicaid: Under the EHR Incentive Program (Meaningful Use) Final Rule, hospitals which are eligible to receive incentive payments include acute care hospitals and children's hospitals

Eligible professional (EP)—Medicare Fee For Service (FFS): MDs, DOs, dentists, dental surgeons, podiatrists, optometrists, and chiropractors who are legally authorized to practice their profession under state law

Eligible professional (EP)—Medicare Advantage (MA): Must furnish at least 20 hrs/week patient care and be employed by a qualifying MA organization or must be employed by a partner of an entity that through contract with the MA organization furnishes at least 80 percent of the entity's Medicare patient care services to enrollees of the qualifying MA organization

Eligible professional (EP)—Medicaid: Physicians, nurse practitioners, certified nurse midwives, dentists, or physician assistants working in a federally qualified health center or rural health clinic that is also led by a PA

Eligibility date: The date on which a member of an insured group may apply for insurance

Eligibility period: The period of time following the eligibility date (usually 31 days) during which a member of an insured group may apply for insurance without evidence of insurability

ELISA: *See* **enzyme-linked immunosorbent assay**

E/M: evaluation and management

E/M coding: *See* **evaluation and management codes**

EMDS: *See* **Essential Medical Data Set**

Emergency and trauma care: The medical-surgical care provided to individuals whose injuries or illnesses require urgent care to address conditions that could be life threatening or disabling if not treated immediately

Emergency access procedures: A process required by HIPAA that provides access in an emergency situation to healthcare providers even if they do not normally have access to the information

Emergency Care Research Institute: *See* **ECRI**

Emergency department: An organized hospital-based facility providing unscheduled episodic services to patients who present for immediate medical attention

Emergency Maternal and Infant Care Program (EMIC): The federal medical program that provides obstetrical and infant care to dependents of active-duty military personnel in the four lowest pay grades

Emergency Medical Treatment and Active Labor Act (EMTALA): A 1986 law enacted as part of the Consolidated Omnibus Reconciliation Act largely to combat "patient dumping"—the transferring, discharging, or refusal to treat indigent emergency department patients because of their inability to pay

Emergency mode operation plan: A plan that defines the processes and controls that will be followed until the operations are fully restored; *Also called* **crisis management plan**

Emergency patient: A patient who is admitted to the emergency services department of a hospital for the diagnosis and treatment of a condition that requires immediate medical, dental, or allied health services in order to sustain life or to prevent critical consequences

Emergency preparedness: A state of readiness to react to an emergency situation

Emergency services: Immediate evaluation and therapy rendered in urgent clinical conditions and sustained until the patient can be referred to his or her personal practitioner for further care

EMG: electromyogram

EMIC: *See* **Emergency Maternal and Infant Care Program**

EMPI: *See* **enterprise master patient index**

Empiricism: The quality of being based on observed and validated evidence

Employee orientation: The process in which employees are introduced to an organization and a new job

Employee record: The document in which an employee's information relating to job performance and so on is kept

Employee Retirement Income Security Act of 1974 (ERISA): An act that sets minimum standards for most voluntarily established pension and health plans in private industry to provide protection for individuals in these plans

Employer-based self-insurance: An umbrella term used to describe health plans that are funded directly by employers to provide coverage for their employees exclusively in which employers establish accounts to cover their employees' medical expenses and retain control over the funds but bear the risk of paying claims greater than their estimates

Employer identification number (EIN): The federal tax identification number of a business, designated in HIPAA as the standard identifier for employers

Employment-at-will: Concept that employees can be fired at any time and for almost any reason based on the idea that employees can quit at any time and for any reason

Employment contract: A legal and binding agreement of terms related to an individual's work, such as hours, pay, or benefits

Empowerment: The condition of having the environment and resources to perform a job independently

EMR: *See* **electronic medical record**

EMTALA: *See* **Emergency Medical Treatment and Active Labor Act**

Enabling technologies: Any newly developed equipment that facilitates data gathering or information processing not possible previously

Encoded: Converted into code

Encoder: Specialty software used to facilitate the assignment of diagnostic and procedural codes according to the rules of the coding system

Encounter: The professional, direct personal contact between a patient and a physician or other person who is authorized by state licensure law and, if applicable, by medical staff bylaws to order or furnish healthcare services for the diagnosis or treatment of the patient; face-to-face contact between a patient and a provider who has primary responsibility for assessing and treating the condition of the patient at a given contact and exercises independent judgment in the care of the patient

Encryption: The process of transforming text into an unintelligible string of characters that can be transmitted via communications media with a high degree of security and then decrypted when it reaches a secure destination

Ending: The transition process that begins with the recognition that the old way of doing things is being terminated

End product: The final result(s) of healthcare services in terms of the patient's expectations, needs, and quality of life, which may be positive and appropriate or negative and diminishing

End-stage renal disease: The point at which there is permanent kidney failure and dialysis or transplant are the only two options of treatment left for a patient

Enforcement rule: A rule that created standardized procedures and substantive requirements for investigating complaints and imposing civil monetary penalties (CMPs) for HIPAA violations, as well as a uniform compliance and enforcement mechanism that addresses all of the administrative simplification regulations, including privacy, security, and transactions and code sets

Enterprise content and record management (ECRM): Convergence of enterprisewide content management

(ECM) and electronic record management (ERM) that provides functionality for managing all content across its lifecycle according to legal, regulatory, and operational requirements. Ability to imbed content classification and retention rules, and integrate with collaboration tools

Enterprise master patient index (EMPI): An index that provides access to multiple repositories of information from overlapping patient populations that are maintained in separate systems and databases

Enterprise resource planning (ERP): The use of software tools to automate tasks and track data generated by specific departments (primarily finance, inventory, and human resources) in order to optimize resource utilization

Enterprisewide content management (ECM): Consists of a cluster of technologies that manage the enterprise's unstructured intellectual substance of its documents and records, such as symbol, image, video, and audio data

Entity: An individual person, group, or organization

Entity authentication: The corroboration that an entity is who it claims to be

Entity relationship diagram (ERD): A specific type of data modeling used in conceptual data modeling and the logical-level modeling of relational databases

Environmental assessment: A thorough review of the internal and external conditions in which an organization operates

Environmental Protection Agency (EPA) Substance Registry System (SRS): Interoperability standard for chemicals that provides a common basis for identification of chemicals, biological organisms, and other substances listed in EPA regulations and data systems

Environmental scanning: A systematic and continuous effort to search for important cues about how the world is changing outside and inside the organization

Enzyme-linked immunosorbent assay (ELISA): A test used to detect the presence of HIV antibody and antigen in both blood and bodily fluids

EOB: *See* **explanation of benefits**

EOC reimbursement: *See* **episode-of-care reimbursement**

EP: *See* **eligible provider**

EPA: *See* **Equal Pay Act of 1963**

EPA SRS: *See* **Environmental Protection Agency Substance Registry System**

ePHI: *See* **Electronic Protected Health Information**

Epidemiological data: Data used to reveal disease trends within a specific population

Epidemiological studies: Studies that are concerned with finding the causes and effects of diseases and conditions

Episode: The 60-day unit of payment for the home health prospective payment system

Episode of care: 1. A period of relatively continuous medical care performed by healthcare professionals in relation to a particular clinical problem or situation 2. One or more healthcare services given by a provider during a specific period of relatively continuous care in relation to a particular health or medical problem or situation 3. In home health, all home care services and nonroutine medical supplies delivered to a patient during a 60-day period; the episode of care is the unit of payment under the home health prospective payment system (HHPPS)

Episode-of-care (EOC) reimbursement: A category of payments made as lump sums to providers for all healthcare services delivered to a patient for a specific illness and/or over a specified time period; *Also called* **bundled payments** because they include multiple services and may include multiple providers of care

EPO: *See* **exclusive provider organization**

e-prescribing (e-Rx): *See* **electronic prescribing**

EPSS: *See* **Electronic Performance Support System**

Equal Employment Opportunity Act: The 1972 amendment to the Civil Rights Act of 1964 prohibiting discrimination in the workplace on the basis of age, gender, race, color, religion, sex, or national origin

Equal Pay Act of 1963 (EPA): The federal legislation that requires equal pay for men and women who perform substantially the same work

Equipment: A long-term (fixed) asset account representing depreciable items owned by the organization that have value over multiple fiscal years (for example, the historical cost of a CT scanner is recorded in an equipment account); *See* **fixed assets**

Equity: Securities that are shared in the ownership of the organization

Equity financing: The retained earnings or profits generated by an organization

ER: emergency room

ER modeling: A term used in the context of information management and technology to describe a graphic technique used for the understanding and organization of data independent of actual implementation of a database

ERA: *See* **electronic remittance advice**

ERD: *See* **entity relationship diagram**

Ergonomics: A discipline of functional design associated with the employee in relationship to his or her work environment, including equipment, workstation, and office furniture adaptation to accommodate the employee's unique physical requirements so as to facilitate efficacy of work functions

ERISA: *See* **Employee Retirement Income Security Act of 1974**

ERM/COLD: *See* **electronic record management**

ERP: *See* **enterprise resource planning**

Error: Act involving an unintentional deviation from truth or accuracy

E-Rx: *See* **electronic prescribing**

ESA: *See* **electronic signature authentication**

ESI: *See* **electronically stored information**

Esprit de corps: Enthusiasm among the members of a group supporting the group's existence

ESRD: end-stage renal disease

Essential Medical Data Set (EMDS): A recommended data set designed to create a health history for an individual patient treated in an emergency service

Established Name for Active Ingredients and FDA Unique Ingredient Identifier (UNII) Codes: Interoperability standard for active ingredients in medications

Established patient: A patient who has received professional services from the physician or another physician of the same specialty in the same practice group within the past three years

Ethernet: A popular protocol (format) for transmitting data in local-area networks

Ethical decision making: The process of requiring everyone to consider the perspectives of others, even when they do not agree with them

Ethicist: An individual trained in the application of ethical theories and principles to problems that cannot be easily solved because of conflicting values, perspectives, and options for action

Ethics: A field of study that deals with moral principles, theories, and values; in healthcare, a formal decision-making process for dealing with the competing perspectives and obligations of the people who have an interest in a common problem

Ethics training: The act of teaching others about moral principles, theories, and values

Ethnic group: The cultural group with which the patient identifies by means of either recorded family data or personal preference

Ethnicity: A category in the Uniform Hospital Discharge Data Set that describes a patient's cultural or racial background

Ethnography: A method of observational research that investigates culture in naturalistic settings using both qualitative and quantitative approaches

Etiologic diagnosis: Underlying cause or origin of a problem that leads to a certain diagnosis or condition

Etiology axis: The cause of a disease or injury

European Committee for Standardization: A business facilitator in Europe, removing trade barriers for European industry and consumers; through its services it provides a platform for the development of European Standards and other technical specifications.

Evaluation and management (E/M) codes: Current Procedural Terminology codes that describe patient encounters with healthcare professionals for assessment counseling and other routine healthcare services

Evaluation and management (E/M) services: The history, examination, and medical decision-making services that physicians must perform in evaluating and treating patients in all healthcare settings

Evaluation research: A design of research that examines the effectiveness of policies, programs, or organizations

Evidence: The means by which the facts of a case are proved or disproved

Evidence-based clinical practice guideline: Explicit statement that guides clinical decision making and has been systematically developed from scientific evidence and clinical expertise to answer clinical questions;

systematic use of guidelines is termed evidence-based medicine

Evidence-based management: A management system in which practices based on research evidence will be effective and produce the outcomes they claim

Evidence-based medicine: Healthcare services based on clinical methods that have been thoroughly tested through controlled, peer-reviewed biomedical studies

Evidence-based practices: Services that use decision support systems and best practices in medicine rather than relying on subjective information

Evidence of insurability: Statement or proof of a health status necessary to obtain healthcare insurance, especially private healthcare insurance

Exacerbation: To make more violent, bitter, or severe

Examination: The act of evaluating the body to determine the presence or absence of disease

Examination types: The levels of E/M services define four types of examination: problem-focused (an examination that is limited to the affected body area or organ system); expanded problem-focused (an examination of the affected body area or organ system and other symptomatic or related organ systems); detailed (an extended examination of the affected body area[s] and other symptomatic or related organ systems); and comprehensive (a complete single-system specialty examination or a general multisystem examination)

Excision: Cutting out or off, without replacement, a portion of a body part

Excisional breast biopsy: A breast biopsy that includes the removal of the entire lesion, whether benign or malignant

Exclusion: A specified condition or circumstance listed in an insurance policy for which the policy will not provide benefits; *Also called* **impairment rider**

Exclusive provider organization (EPO): Hybrid managed care organization that provides benefits to subscribers only when healthcare services are performed by network providers; sponsored by self-insured (self-funded) employers or associations and exhibits characteristics of both health maintenance organizations and preferred provider organizations

Executive dashboard: An information management system providing decision makers with regularly updated information on an organization's key strategic measures

Executive decision support system: *See* **executive information system**

Executive information system (EIS): An information system designed to combine financial and clinical information for use in the management of business affairs of a healthcare organization; *Also called* **executive decision support system**

Executive management: The managerial level of an organization that is primarily responsible for setting the organization's future direction and establishing its strategic plan while maintaining the organization's mission and vision

Executive manager: A senior manager who oversees a broad functional area or group of departments or services, sets the organization's future direction, and monitors the organization's operations in those areas

Executive sponsor: An individual who helps a team leader keep the team on track and sometimes ensures that the team obtains the organizational support required to accomplish its goal

Exempt employees: Specific groups of employees who are identified as not being covered by some or all of the provisions of the Fair Labor Standards Act

Exit conference: A meeting that closes a site visit during which the surveyors representing an accrediting organization summarize their findings and explain any deficiencies that have been identified; at this time, the leadership of the organization also is allowed an opportunity to discuss the surveyors' perspectives or to provide additional information related to any deficiencies the surveyors intend to cite in their final reports

Exit interview: The final meeting an employee has with his or her employer before leaving the organization

Expectancy theory of motivation: Proposes that one's efforts will result in the attainment of desired performance goals

Expectations: The characteristics that customers want to be evident in a healthcare product, service, or outcome

Expenses: Amounts that are charged as costs by an organization to the current year's activities of operation

Experimental research: 1. A research design used to establish cause and effect 2. A controlled investigation in which subjects are assigned randomly to groups that experience carefully controlled interventions that are manipulated by the experimenter according to a strict protocol; *Also called* **experimental study**

Experimental study: *See* **experimental research**

Experimental (study) group: A group of participants in which the exposure status of each participant is determined and the individuals are followed forward to determine the effects of the exposure

Expert decision support system: A decision support system that uses a set of rules or encoded concepts to construct a reasoning process

Expert knowledge-based information system: Information system that assists physicians and other healthcare providers in the diagnosis and treatment of a patient

Expert system (ES): A type of information system that supports the work of professionals engaged in the development or evaluation of complex activities that require high-level knowledge in a well-defined and usually limited area

Expert witness: An individual called to testify in a case based on their expertise in a certain subject

Explanation of benefits (EOB): A statement issued to the insured and the healthcare provider by an insurer to explain the services provided, amounts billed, and payments made by a health plan. *See* **payer remittance report**

Explicit knowledge: Documents, databases, and other types of recorded and documented information

Exploding charges: Charges for items that must be reported separately but are used together, such as interventional radiology imaging and injection procedures

Exploratory research: A research design used because a problem has not been clearly defined or its scope is unclear

Expressed consent: The spoken or written permission granted by a patient to a healthcare provider that allows the provider to perform medical or surgical services

Extended care facility: A healthcare facility licensed by applicable state or local law to offer room and board, skilled nursing by a full-time registered nurse, intermediate care, or a combination of levels on a 24-hour basis over a long period of time

Extensible markup language (XML): A standardized computer language that allows the interchange of data as structured text

External cause of injury code: *See* **E code**

External customers: Individuals from outside the organization who receive products or services from within the organization

External data: Data coming from outside the facility that can be used to compare the facility with other similar facilities

External review (audit): A performance or quality review conducted by a third-party payer or consultant hired for the purpose; *See* **audit**

External validity: An attribute of a study's design that allows its findings to be applied to other groups

Extirpation: Taking or cutting out solid matter from a body part. The objective is to remove solid matter such as a foreign body, thrombus, or calculus from the body part

Extracapsular lens extraction: The surgical removal of the front portion and nucleus of the lens, leaving the posterior capsule in place. A posterior chamber intraocular lens is generally inserted after this procedure

Extraction: Pulling or stripping out or off a portion of a body part by the use of force

Extraneous variable: *See* **confounding variable**

Extranet: A system of connections of private Internet networks outside an organization's firewall that uses Internet technology to enable collaborative applications among enterprises

Extreme immaturity: A condition referring to a newborn with a birth weight of fewer than 1,000 grams and/or gestation of fewer than 28 completed weeks

Face page: Introductory material on a grant proposal, similar to a title page

Face sheet: Usually the first page of the health record, which contains patient identification, demographics, date of admission, insurance coverage or payment source, referral information, hospital stay dates, physician information, and discharge information, as well as the name of the responsible party, emergency and additional contacts, and the resident's diagnoses

Face validity: The extent to which a study's findings can be generalized to other people or groups

Facilities, health: Buildings, including physical plant, equipment, and supplies, necessary in the provision of health services (for example, hospitals, nursing homes, and ambulatory care centers)

Facilities management: The functional oversight of a healthcare organization's physical plant to ensure operational efficiency in an environment that is safe for patients, staff, and visitors

Facility access controls: HIPAA Security Rule requirement that policies and procedures limit physical access to authorized staff to the data centers where the hardware and software for the electronic information systems are held

Facility-based registry: A registry that includes only cases from a particular type of healthcare facility, such as a hospital or clinic

Facility coding: In relationship to hospital outpatient services, facility coding represents the services provided by the hospital in the form of space, equipment, staff, and supplies. This coding involves the use of ICD-9-CM diagnosis codes, CPT procedure codes, and HCPCS procedure codes and is reported to payors on the CMS-1450 or UB004 claim form, or the electronic equivalent

Facility directory: A directory of patients being treated in a healthcare facility

Facility identification: A unique universal identification number across data systems for a facility

Facility quality indicator profile: A report based on the data gathered during the Minimum Data Set for Long-Term Care that indicates what proportion of the facility's residents have deficits in each area of assessment during the reporting period and, specifically, which residents have which deficits; the profile also provides data comparing the facility's current status with a preestablished comparison group

Facility specific index: Databases established by healthcare facilities to meet their individual, specific needs for customer care or other reporting requirements. These indexes make it possible to retrieve health records in a variety of ways including by disease, physician, operation, or other data element. Prior to computerization in healthcare, these indexes were kept on cards. Today, most are compiled from databases routinely developed by the facility

Facility-specific system: A computer information system developed exclusively to meet the needs of one healthcare organization

Facsimile: A machine that allows the remote transmission of text and graphics through telephone lines or a communication sent via this method; *Also called* **fax**

FACTA: *See* **Fair and Accurate Credit Transaction Act**

Factor analysis: A statistical technique in which a large number of variables are summarized and reduced to a smaller number based on similar relationships among those variables

Factor comparison method: A complex quantitative method of job evaluation that combines elements of both the ranking and point methods

FAHIMA: Fellow of the American Health Information Management Association; *See* **Fellowship Program**

Failed/missed appointment policy: Policy that tracks appointments that are canceled or missed. A failed/missed appointment policy should state the required documentation of information concerning the missed appointment

Failure Mode Effect and Criticality Assessment (FMECA): A methodology for determining the cause of sentinel events

Fair and Accurate Credit Transaction Act (FACTA): Law passed in 2003 that contains provisions and requirements to reduce identity theft

Fair Labor Standards Act of 1938 (FLSA): The federal legislation that sets the minimum wage and overtime payment regulations

False Claims Act: 1. Legislation passed during the Civil War that prohibits contractors from making a false claim to a governmental program; used to reinforce the prevention of healthcare fraud and abuse 2. An American federal law that allows individuals to file actions against federal contractors who are accused of submitting fraudulent claims

False cost reports: A way of increasing Medicare payments inappropriately by submitting inaccurate financial reports

Family and Medical Leave Act of 1993 (FMLA): The federal legislation that allows full-time employees time off from work (up to 12 weeks) to care for themselves or their family members with the assurance of an equivalent position upon return to work

Family numbering: A filing system, sometimes used in clinic settings, in which an entire family is assigned one number

FASB: *See* **Financial Accounting Standards Board**

Favorable variance: The positive difference between the budgeted amount and the actual amount of a line item, that is, when actual revenue exceeds budget or actual expenses are less than budget

Fax: *See* **facsimile**

Faxing policy: A policy that outlines the steps to take for faxing individually identifiable health information and business records and usually limits what information may be faxed

Fax on demand: A service in which a user may select from a list of available fax sources by keying the corresponding number of a fax title or from multiple fax messages via a 12-digit telephone keypad

FCA: *See* **False Claims Act**

FDA: *See* **Food and Drug Administration**

Feasibility: The realistic likelihood of an evaluation's success given the available time, resources, and expertise

Feasibility study: A study that looks at factors affecting an issue's ability to generate the necessary cash flows to meet principal and interest requirements

FECA: *See* **Federal Employees' Compensation Act**

Federal Anti-Kickback Statute: A statute that establishes criminal penalties for individuals and entities that knowingly and willfully offer, pay, solicit or receive remuneration in order to induce business for which payment may be made under any federal healthcare program

Federal Employees' Compensation Act (FECA): The legislation enacted in 1916 to mandate workers' compensation for civilian federal employees, whose coverage includes lost wages, medical expenses, and survivors' benefits

Federal Food, Drug and Cosmetic Act (FFDCA): The basic authority intended to ensure that foods are pure and wholesome, safe to eat, and produced under sanitary conditions; that drugs and devices are safe and effective for their intended uses; that cosmetics are safe and made from appropriate ingredients; and that all labeling and packaging is truthful, informative and not deceptive

Federal Health Architecture (FHA): E-Government Line of Business initiative managed by the Office of the National Coordinator for Health IT. FHA was formed to coordinate health IT activities among the more than 20 federal agencies that provide health and healthcare services to citizens

Federal Physician Self-Referral Statute (Stark): Originally a part of the Omnibus Budget Reconciliation Act of 1989, it is a law that prohibits physicians from ordering designated health services for Medicare (and to some extent Medicaid) patients from entities with which the physician, or an immediate family member, has a financial relationship; *Also called* the Stark Law

Federal poverty level (FPL): The income qualification threshold established by the federal government for certain government entitlement programs

Federal Register: The daily publication of the US Government Printing Office that reports all changes in regulations and federally mandated standards, including HCPCS and ICD-9-CM codes

Federal Rules of Civil Procedure (FRCP): Rules established by the US Supreme Court setting the "rules of the road" and procedures for federal court cases. FRCP were amended in 2006 to include electronic records and continue to be very important as benchmarks in how these records can be used in courts, not only federal, but state and other courts as well. Record custodianship is widely discussed within the FRCP

Federal Rules of Evidence (FRE): Rules established by the US Supreme Court guiding the introduction and use of evidence in federal court proceedings that are an important benchmark for state and other courts. FRE governs what and how electronic records may be used, and the roles of record custodianship

Federal Trade Commission (FTC): An independent federal agency tasked with dealing with two areas of economics in the United States: consumer protection and issues having to do with competition in business

Fee: Price assigned to a unit of medical or health service, such as a visit to a physician or a day in a hospital; may be unrelated to the actual cost of providing the service; *See* **charge**

Fee schedule: A list of healthcare services and procedures (usually CPT/HCPCS codes) and the charges associated with them developed by a third-party payer to represent the approved payment levels for a given insurance plan; *Also called* **table of allowances**

Feeder system: An information system that operates independently but provides data to other systems such as an EHR; *Also called* **source system**

Fee-for-service basis: *See* **fee-for-service (FFS) reimbursement**

Fee-for-service (FFS) reimbursement: A method of reimbursement through which providers retrospectively receive payment based on either billed charges for services provided or on annually updated fee schedules; *Also called* **fee-for-service basis**

Fellowship Program: Program of earned recognition for AHIMA members who have made significant and sustained contributions to the HIM profession through meritorious service, excellence in professional practice, education, and advancement of the profession through innovation and knowledge sharing

Felony: A serious crime such as murder, larceny, rape, or assault for which punishment is usually severe

FEP: *See* **Blue Cross and Blue Shield Federal Employee Program**

Fetal autopsy rate: The number of autopsies performed on intermediate and late fetal deaths for a given time period divided by the total number of intermediate and late fetal deaths for the same time period

Fetal death: The death of a product of human conception before its complete expulsion or extraction from the mother regardless of the duration of the pregnancy; *See* **stillbirth**

Fetal death rate: A proportion that compares the number of intermediate and/or late fetal deaths to the total number of live births and intermediate or late fetal deaths during the same period of time

FFDCA: *See* **Federal Food, Drug and Cosmetic Act**

FFS reimbursement: *See* **fee-for-service reimbursement**; **traditional fee-for-service reimbursement**

FHA: *See* **Federal Health Architecture**

FI: *See* **fiscal intermediary**

Fidelity: A quality closely aligned with honesty; includes keeping promises, honoring contracts and agreements, and telling the truth

Field notes: Notes that are recorded either immediately after the observation or during short breaks between observations

File transfer protocol (FTP): A communications protocol that enables users to copy or move files between computer systems

FIM: *See* **functional independence measure**

Final note: A note becomes finalized either through attestation and system requirement or after a defined period of time, per organizational policies and procedures, applicable rules and regulations, and/or medical staff bylaws

Final signature: The process of applying the responsible provider's electronic signature to documentation. Once applied, the documentation is considered complete

Financial accounting: The mechanism that organizations use to fully comprehend and communicate their financial activities

Financial Accounting Standards Board (FASB): An independent organization that sets accounting standards for businesses in the private sector

Financial data: The data collected for the purpose of managing the assets and expenses of a business (for example, a healthcare organization, a product line); in healthcare, data derived from the charge generation documentation associated with the activities of care and then aggregated by specific customer grouping for financial analysis

Financial indicators: A set of measures designed to routinely monitor the current financial status of a healthcare organization or of one of its constituent parts

Financial information system: The accounting and financial programs and data necessary for running a healthcare facility

Financial transaction: The exchange of goods or services for payment or the promise of payment

Firewall: A computer system or a combination of systems that provides a security barrier or supports an access control policy between two networks or between a network and any other traffic outside the network

Fiscal intermediary (FI): An organization that contracts with the Centers for Medicare and Medicaid Services to serve as the financial agent between providers and the federal government in the local administration of Medicare Part A or Part B claims; usually, but not necessarily, an insurance company

Fiscal year: Any consecutive 12-month period an organization uses as its accounting period

Fishbone diagram: A performance improvement tool used to identify or classify the root causes of a problem or condition and to display the root causes graphically; *See also* **cause-and-effect diagram**

Fixed assets: Long-term assets; *See also* **capital assets**; **property, plant, and equipment**

Fixed budget: A type of budget based on expected capacity with no consideration of potential variations

Fixed costs: Resources expended that do not vary with the activity of the organization (for example, mortgage expense does not vary with patient volume)

Flash drive: A small, portable storage device with multi-gigabyte capacity that connects to a computer via a universal serial bus (USB) connection; also known by several other names, such as jump drive, thumb drive, and others

Flat fee systems: A predefined amount paid for a unit of service

Flat-panel display: The technology using liquid crystal display or other low-emission substances, once found primarily on laptops and now being used for desktop monitors, large-screen wall monitors, and high-density television

Flexibility of approach: Condition under HIPAA Security Rule in which a covered entity can adopt security protection measures that are appropriate for its organization

Flexible budget: A type of budget that is based on multiple levels of projected productivity (actual productivity triggers the levels to be used as the year progresses)

Flexible work schedule: *See* **flextime**

Flextime: A work schedule that gives employees some choice in the pattern of their work hours, usually around a core of midday hours

Flex years: A work arrangement in which employees are paid over a 12-month period, but work less than 12 months

Float employee: An employee who is not assigned to a particular shift, function, or unit and who may fill in as needed in cases of standard employee absence or vacation

Flow chart: A graphic tool that uses standard symbols to visually display detailed information, including time and distance, of the sequential flow of work of an individual or a product as it progresses through a process

Flow process chart: *See* **flow chart**

FLSA: *See* **Fair Labor Standards Act of 1938**

FMECA: *See* **Failure Mode Effect and Criticality Assessment**

FMLA: *See* **Family and Medical Leave Act of 1993**

Focus: An organized form of charting narrative notes in which nursing terminology is used to explain the resident's health status and resulting nursing data, action, and response

Focus group: A group of approximately 6–12 subjects, usually experts in the particular area of study, brought together to discuss a specific topic using the focused interview method, usually with a moderator who is not on the research team

Focused interview: A type of interview used when the researcher wants to collect a more in-depth, heartier type of information not obtainable from closed-ended questions

Focused review: A process whereby a health record is analyzed to gather specific information about the diagnoses, treatments, or providers

Focused study: A study in which a researcher orally questions and conducts discussions with members of a group

FOIA: *See* **Freedom of Information Act of 1967**

Food and Drug Administration (FDA): The federal agency responsible for controlling the sale and use of pharmaceuticals, biological products, medical devices, food, cosmetics, and products that emit radiation, including the licensing of medications for human use; *See* **Federal Food, Drug and Cosmetic Act**

Food and drug interactions: Unexpected conditions that result from the physiologic incompatibility of therapeutic drugs and food consumed by a patient

Force-field analysis: A performance improvement tool used to identify specific drivers of, and barriers to, an organizational change so that positive factors can be reinforced and negative factors reduced

Forecast: To calculate or predict some future event or condition through study and analysis of available pertinent data

Forecast budget: A budgeting approach that simply divides the amount budgeted by the number of months in the fiscal period

Foreign key: A key attribute used to link a column or data point in one table to the column or data point in another table

Formative evaluation: Evaluations that measure or assess improvement in delivery methods with regard to technology used; quality of implementation of a new process or technology; information about the organizational placement of a given process; type of personnel involved in a program; or other important factors such as the procedures, source, and type of inputs

Forming: The first of four steps in assembling a functional team

Forms automation: The process of automating a paper form in a database so that the form can be printed from multiple locations throughout the organization and included within the health record

Forms management policy: A policy that outlines the process for the creation of new forms

Formulary: A listing of drugs, classified by therapeutic category or disease class; in some health plans, providers are limited to prescribing only drugs listed on the plan's formulary. The selection of items to be included in the formulary is based on objective evaluations of their relative therapeutic merits, safety, and cost

For-profit organization: The tax status assigned to business entities that are owned by one or more individuals or organizations and that earn revenues in excess of expenditures that are subsequently paid out to the owners or stockholders

Foundation model: *See* **independent practice organization**

Fourteen principles of management: Henri Fayol's key points in the formulation of the administrative approach to management

42 CFR Part 2: Federal confidentiality regulations governing and protecting records of clients receiving treatment for alcohol and drug abuse–related conditions

FPL: *See* **federal poverty level**

Fraction: One or more parts of a whole

Fragmentation: Breaking solid matter in a body part into pieces

Frame data: *See* **motion video**

Fraud: 1. An intentional misrepresentation of facts to deceive or mislead in order to unjustly gain from another party 2. Intentionally making a claim for payment that one knows to be false

FRCP: *See* **Federal Rules of Civil Procedure**

FRE: *See* **Federal Rules of Evidence**

Freedom of Information Act of 1967 (FOIA): The federal law, applicable only to federal agencies, through which individuals can seek access to information without the authorization of the person to whom the information applies

Freestanding facility: In Medicare terminology, an entity that furnishes healthcare services to beneficiaries and is not integrated with any other entity as a main provider, a department of a provider, or a provider-based entity

Free-text data: Data that are narrative in nature

Frequency distribution: A table or graph that displays the number of times (frequency) a particular observation occurs

Frequency distribution table: A table consisting of a set of classes or categories along with the numerical counts that correspond to nominal and ordinal data

Frequency polygon: A type of line graph that represents a frequency distribution

Front-end processes: The billing processes associated with preregistration, prebooking, scheduling, and registration activities that collect patient demographic and insurance information, perform verification of patient insurance, and determine medical necessity

Front-end speech recognition: The specific use of speech recognition technology in an environment where the recognition process occurs in real time (or near-real time) as dictation takes place

FTE: *See* **full-time equivalent**

FTP: *See* **file transfer protocol**

Full-time employee: An employee who works 40 hours per week, 80 hours per two-week period, or 8 hours per day

Full-time equivalent (FTE): A statistic representing the number of full-time employees as calculated by the reported number of hours worked by all employees, including part-time and temporary, during a specific time period

Fully Specified Name: In SNOMED CT, the unique text assigned to a concept that completely describes that concept

Function: A term used to describe an entity or activity that involves a single healthcare department, service area, or discipline

Functional independence measure (FIM): Measure used to evaluate the level of independence of patients in long-term acute-care (LTCH) settings where the focus of care is on extensive rehabilitation of the patient. FIM includes 18 items that are scored on a scale of 1 to 7, with 1 being the most dependent and 7 being the most independent. Total scores range between 18 and 126. FIM scores can be used as outcome measures by LTCHs

Functional independent assessment tool: Standardized tool to measure the severity of patients' impairments in rehabilitation settings. The tool captures characteristics that reflect the functional status of patients. Patients with lower scores on the tool have less independence and need more assistance than patients with higher scores

Functional needs assessment: An assessment that describes the key capabilities or application requirements for achieving the benefits of the EHR as the organization has envisioned it

Functional requirement: A statement that describes the processes a computer system should perform to derive the technical specifications, or desired behavior, of a system

Functional status: A commonly used measure of a patient's mental and/or physical abilities measuring the patient's ability to perform the activities of daily living

Functional status domain: A classification made up of six activities of daily living, including upper and lower body dressing, bathing, toileting, transferring, and moving

Function axis: Physiological or chemical disorders and alterations resulting from a disease or injury

Functionality standards: Standards that define the components that an electronic health record needs to support the functions for which it is designed; HL7 standards are an example

Fund balance: In a not-for-profit setting, the entity's net assets or resources remaining after subtracting liabilities that are owed; in a for-profit organization, the owner's equity

Fusion: Joining together portions of an articular body part rendering the articular body part immobile. Only performed on joints

Future value: The total dollar amount of an investment at a later point in time, including any earned or implied interest

Fuzzy logic: An analytic technique used in data mining to handle imprecise concepts

GAAP: *See* **generally accepted accounting principles**

GAAS: *See* **generally accepted auditing standards**

GAF: *See* **geographic adjustment factor**

Galen Common Reference Model (Galen CRM): A computer-based clinical terminology developed in Europe for representing medical concepts

Gantt chart: A graphic tool used to plot tasks in project management that shows the duration of project tasks and overlapping tasks

Gap analysis: 1. A review of the collected literature and data to assess whether gaps exist 2. Advice for those conducting the literature review on additional literature and data sources missed

Garnishment: A method of collecting a monetary award in which a certain percentage of the defendant's wages are routinely set aside and paid to the plaintiff toward full satisfaction of the judgment

GASB: *See* **Government Accounting Standards Board**

Gatekeeper: The healthcare provider or entity responsible for determining the healthcare services a patient or client may access; for instance, a primary care physician, a utilization review or case management agency, or a managed care organization

GEMs: *See* **General Equivalence Mappings**

Gender: The biological sex of the patient as recorded at the start of care

Gender rule: A method of determining which insurance company is the primary carrier for dependents when both parents carry insurance on them. The rule states that the insurance for the male of the household is considered primary

General consent: *See* **general consent to treatment**

General consent to treatment: A consent signed upon admission to the facility that allows the clinical staff to provide care and treatment for the resident and that usually includes the resident's agreement to pay for the services provided by the facility, to assign insurance benefits to the facility, and to allow the facility to obtain or release health records for payment purposes; *Also called* **general consent**

General Equivalence Mappings (GEMs): A program created to facilitate the translation between ICD-9-CM and ICD-10-CM/PCS

General health record documentation policy: A policy that outlines documentation practices within the facility

General interview guide: An outline or checklist of issues that the researcher can use for interviews that are a bit more structured than the informal conversational interview, often used with very long interviews that are audiotaped so the researcher has time to focus on the interview process

General jurisdiction: Courts that hear more serious criminal cases or civil cases that involve large amounts of money; may hear all matters of state law except for those cases that must be heard in courts of special jurisdiction

General ledger: A master list of individual revenue and expense accounts maintained by an organization

General ledger (G/L) key: The two- or three-digit number in the chargemaster that assigns each item to a particular section of the general ledger in a healthcare facility's accounting section

Generalizability: The ability to apply research results, data, or observations to groups not originally under study

Generally accepted accounting principles (GAAP): An accepted set of accounting principles or standards, and recognized procedures central to financial accounting and reporting

Generally accepted auditing standards (GAAS): The way in which organizations record and report financial transactions so that financial information is consistent between organizations

General Rules: HIPAA data security provisions that provide the objective and scope for the HIPAA Privacy Rule and Security Rule

Generic: Once a patent for a brand name expires, other manufacturers may copy the drug and release it under its pharmaceutical or "generic" name

Generic device group: The actual nomenclature or naming level by which a product or a group of similar products can be classified in the Global Medical Dictionary Nomenclature using a selected generic descriptor and its unique code

Generic screening: *See* **occurrence screening**

Genetic algorithms: Optimization techniques that can be used to improve other data-mining algorithms so that they derive the best model for a given set of data

Geographic adjustment factor (GAF): Adjustment to the national standardized Medicare fee schedule relative value components used to account for differences in the cost of practicing medicine in different geographic areas of the country

Geographic information system (GIS): A decision support system that is capable of assembling, storing, manipulating, and displaying geographically referenced data and information

Geographic practice cost index (GPCI): An index developed by the Centers for Medicare and Medicaid Services to measure the differences in resource costs among fee schedule areas compared to the national average in the three components of the relative value unit (RVU): physician work, practice expenses, and malpractice coverage; separate GPCIs exist for each element of the RVU and are used to adjust the RVUs, which are national averages, to reflect local costs

Geometric mean length of stay (GMLOS): A statistically adjusted value of all cases of a given Medicare severity diagnosis-related group (MS-DRG), allowing for the outliers, transfer cases, and negative outlier cases that would normally skew that data; used to compute hospital reimbursement for transfer cases

Gesture recognition technology: A method of encoding handwritten, print, or cursive characters and of interpreting the characters as words or the intent of the writer

GIS: *See* **geographic information system**

G/L key: *See* **general ledger key**

Global Assessment of Functioning (GAF) Scale: A 100-point tool rating overall psychological, social, and occupational functioning of individuals, excluding physical and environmental impairment

Global Medical Device Nomenclature (GMDN): A collection of internationally recognized terms used to accurately describe and catalog medical devices; in particular, the products used in the diagnosis, prevention, monitoring, treatment, or alleviation of disease or injury in humans

Global package: *See* **surgical package**

Global payment: A form of reimbursement used for radiological and other procedures that combines the professional and technical components of the procedures and disperses payments as lump sums to be distributed between the physician and the healthcare facility

Global payment method: Method of payment in which the third-party payer makes one consolidated payment to cover the services of multiple providers who are treating a single episode of care

Global surgery payment: A payment made for surgical procedures that includes the provision of all healthcare services, from the treatment decision through postoperative patient care

GMDN: *See* **Global Medical Device Nomenclature**

GMLOS: *See* **geometric mean length of stay**

Goal: A specific description of the services or deliverable goods to be provided as the result of a business process

Going concern: An organization that can be assumed to continue indefinitely unless otherwise stated

Gonioscopy: The examination of the angle of the anterior chamber of the eye with a lens, or gonioscope

Good Samaritan statute: State law or statute that protects healthcare providers from liability for not obtaining informed consent before rendering care to adults or minors at the scene of an emergency or accident

Government Accounting Standards Board (GASB): The federal agency that sets the accounting standards to be followed by government entities

GPCI: *See* **geographic practice cost index**

GPWW: *See* **group practice without walls**

Grace period: An amount of time beyond a due date during which a payment may be made without incurring penalties; in healthcare, the specific time (usually 31 days) following the premium due date during which insurance remains in effect and a policyholder may pay the premium without penalty or loss of benefits

Grant: Monetary assistance provided to a facility, university, or individual who will then use this monetary assistance to fully carry out and complete an intended research study

Grantee: Recipient of a research grant, who is responsible for carrying out the research with little or no direct involvement from the granting agency

Granular: Consisting of small components or details

Granularity: Level of detail

Graph: A graphic tool used to show numerical data in a pictorial representation

Graphical user interface (GUI): A style of computer interface in which typed commands are replaced by images that represent tasks (for example, small pictures [icons] that represent the tasks, functions, and programs performed by a software program)

Graphics-based decision support system: A decision support system in which the knowledge base consists primarily of graphical data and the user interface exploits the use of graphical display

Great person theory: The belief that some people have natural (innate) leadership skills

Grievance: A formal, written description of a complaint or disagreement

Grievance management: The policies and procedures used to handle employee complaints

Grievance procedures: The steps employees may follow to seek resolution of disagreements with management on job-related issues

Gross autopsy rate: The number of inpatient autopsies conducted during a given time period divided by the total number of inpatient deaths for the same time period

Gross death rate: The number of inpatient deaths that occurred during a given time period divided by the total number of inpatient discharges, including deaths, for the same time period

Gross patient service revenues: The total amount the healthcare organization earns in full for its services

Ground rules: An agreement concerning attendance, time management, participation, communication, decision making, documentation, room arrangements and cleanup, and so forth, that has been developed by PI team members at the initiation of the team's work

Grounded theory: A theory about what is actually going on instead of what should go on

Group case study: A case study in which the interviews and observations are performed on a group of individuals instead of just one individual

Group health insurance: A prepaid medical plan that covers the healthcare expenses of an organization's full-time, and in some cases, part-time, employees

Group model health maintenance organization: A type of health plan in which an HMO contracts with an independent multispecialty physician group to provide medical services to members of the plan

Group number: Number identifying the employer, association, or other entity that purchases healthcare insurance for the individual members of the group

Group practice: An organization of physicians who share office space and administrative support services to achieve economies of scale; often a clinic or ambulatory care center

Group practice model: A closed-panel health maintenance organization (HMO) in which the HMO contracts with a medical group and reimburses the group on a fee-for-service or capitation basis; *See* **closed panel**; **network model**

Group practice without walls (GPWW): A type of managed care contract that allows physicians to maintain their own offices and share administrative services; *Also called* **clinic without walls (CWW)**

Group process: An intragroup activity of relevance to organizational effectiveness that includes elements such as socialization of new members and conflict resolution

Group therapy: The practice of one therapist providing the same therapeutic services to everyone in the group, in which residents may benefit by observing other residents in the group performing the same activity

Grouper: 1. Computer program that uses specific data elements to assign patients, clients, or residents to groups, categories, or classes 2. A computer software program that automatically assigns prospective payment groups on the basis of clinical codes

Grouping: A system for assigning patients to a classification scheme via a computer software program

Groupthink: An implicit form of group consensus in which openness and effective decision making are sacrificed to conformity

Groupware: An Internet technology that consolidates documents from different information systems within an organization into a tightly integrated workflow

Guarantor: Person who is responsible for paying the bill or guarantees payment for healthcare services; adult patients are often their own guarantors, but parents guarantee payments for the healthcare costs of their children

GUI: *See* **graphical user interface**

H

HAART: *See* **highly active antiretroviral therapy**

Habit: An activity repeated so often that it becomes automatic

Hacker: An individual who bypasses a computer system's access control by taking advantage of system security weaknesses and/or by appropriating the password of an authorized user

Halo effect: A bias that occurs when someone allows certain information to influence a decision disproportionately

Hand-off communication: Communication of patient information between caregivers. The Joint Commission standard 2E recommends that each healthcare organization implement a standardized approach to "hand-off" communications, including an opportunity to ask and respond to questions

Handwritten signature: The most common method for authenticating paper health records

Harassment: The act of bothering or annoying someone repeatedly

Hard code: Referring to a code applied through a healthcare organization's chargemaster

Hard coding: 1. The process of attaching a CPT/HCPCS code to a procedure located on the facility's chargemaster so that the code will automatically be included on the patient's bill 2. Use of the charge description master to code repetitive services

Hard skills: A skill set that includes strategic planning, portfolio management, project planning, resource leveling, issues management, and change control

Hardware: The machines and media used in an information system

Harvard relative value scale study: Research conducted at Harvard University by William Hsiao and Peter Braun on establishing the appropriate relative values for physician services

HAVEN: *See* **Home Assessment Validation and Entry**

Hawthorne effect: A research study that found that novelty, attention, and interpersonal relations have a motivating effect on performance

Hay Guide Chart/Profile Method of Job Evaluation: *See* **Hay method of job evaluation**

Hay method of job evaluation: A modification of the point method of job evaluation that numerically measures the levels of three major compensable factors: know-how, problem-solving ability, and accountability; *Also called* **Hay Guide Chart/Profile Method of Job Evaluation**

HCERA: *See* **Health Care and Education Reconciliation Act of 2010**

HCFA: *See* **Health Care Financing Administration**; now **Centers for Medicare and Medicaid Services (CMS)**

HCFA Common Procedure Coding System (HCPCS): Previous name for the Healthcare Common Procedure Coding System

HCFA-1450: *See* **CMS-1450**

HCFA-1500: *See* **CMS-1500**

HCPCS: *See* **HCFA Common Procedure Coding System; Healthcare Common Procedure Coding System**

HCPCS level I: Current Procedural Terminology (CPT), developed by the American Medical Association

HCPCS level II: Codes not covered by CPT and modifiers that can be used with all levels of codes, developed by the Centers for Medicare and Medicaid Services

HCPCS level III: Codes, often called local codes, developed by local Medicare and/or Medicaid carriers for use in their particular geographic locations; eliminated on December 31, 2003

HCQIA: *See* **Health Care Quality Improvement Act**

HCQIP: *See* **Health Care Quality Improvement Program**

HCRIS: *See* **healthcare provider cost report information system**

HCUP: *See* **Healthcare Cost and Utilization Project**

Health: A state of complete physical, mental, and social well-being and not merely the absence of disease or infirmity

Healthcare claims and payment/advice transaction: An electronic transmission sent by a health plan to a provider's financial representative for the purpose of providing information about payments and/or payment processing and information about the transfer of funds

Healthcare clearinghouse: As defined under HIPAA, a public or private entity (such as a billing service, repricing company, community health management information system, community health information system, or a value-added network) that either processes or facilitates the processing of health information received from another entity in a nonstandard format or containing nonstandard data content into standard data elements or standard transactions; or receives a standard transaction from another entity and processes or facilitates the processing of health information into nonstandard format or nonstandard data content for the receiving entity

Healthcare Common Procedure Coding System (HCPCS): An alphanumeric classification system that identifies healthcare procedures, equipment, and supplies for claim submission purposes; the three levels are as follows: I, Current Procedural Terminology codes, developed by the AMA; II, codes for equipment, supplies, and services not covered by Current Procedural Terminology codes as well as modifiers that can be used with all levels of codes, developed by CMS; and III (eliminated December 31, 2003, to comply with HIPAA), local codes developed by regional Medicare Part B carriers and used to report physicians' services and supplies to Medicare for reimbursement

Healthcare Cost and Utilization Project (HCUP): A group of healthcare databases and related software tools developed through collaboration by the federal government, state governments, and industry to create a national information resource for patient-level healthcare data

Healthcare-covered entity: Defined under the HIPAA Administrative Simplification regulations as any entity that is a healthcare provider that conducts certain transactions in electronic form, a healthcare clearinghouse, or a health plan

Healthcare Facilities Accreditation Program (HFAP): An accreditation program managed by the American Osteopathic Association that offers services to a number of healthcare facilities and services, including laboratories, ambulatory care clinics, ambulatory surgery centers, behavioral health and substance abuse treatment facilities, physical rehabilitation facilities, acute care hospitals, critical access hospitals, and hospitals providing postdoctoral training for osteopathic physicians

Healthcare informatics: The field of information science concerned with the management of all aspects of health data and information through the application of computers and computer technologies; *See* **clinical informatics; informatics; nursing informatics**

Healthcare Information and Management Systems Society (HIMSS): A national membership association that provides leadership in healthcare for the management of technology, information, and change

Healthcare information standards: Guidelines developed to standardize data throughout the healthcare industry (for example, developing uniform terminologies and vocabularies)

Healthcare information system (HIS): A transactional system used in healthcare organizations (for example, patient admitting, accounting, and receivables); *See* **hospital information system**

Healthcare Information Systems Steering Committee: An interdisciplinary team of healthcare professionals generally responsible for developing a strategic information system plan, prioritizing information system projects, and coordinating IS-related projects across the enterprise

Healthcare Information Technology Standards Panel (HITSP): An organization developed under the auspices of the American National Standards Institute (ANSI) to deal with the many issues of privacy and security as the United States Nationwide Health Information Network develops

Healthcare Integrity and Protection Data Bank (HIPDB): A database maintained by the federal government to provide information on fraud-and-abuse findings against US healthcare providers

Healthcare operations: Certain activities undertaken by or on behalf of, a covered entity, including: conducting quality assessment and improvement activities; reviewing the competence or qualifications of healthcare professionals, underwriting, premium rating, and other activities relating to the creation; renewal or replacement of a contract of health insurance or health benefits; conducting or arranging for medical review, legal services, and auditing functions; business planning and development; and business management and general administrative activities of the entity

Healthcare practitioner: A clinical professional who is directly responsible for providing patient services

Healthcare practitioner identification: A unique national identification number assigned to the healthcare practitioner of record for each encounter

Healthcare provider: A provider of diagnostic, medical, and surgical care as well as the services or supplies related to the health of an individual and any other person or organization that issues reimbursement claims or is paid for healthcare in the normal course of business. A provider is legally responsible for the patient's diagnosis and treatment

Healthcare provider cost report information system (HCRIS): A system of Medicare cost report files containing information on provider characteristics, utilization data, and cost and charge data by cost center

Healthcare reengineering: A focus of the healthcare industry whose forces have turned their attention to patient care and cost controls, managed care, integrated delivery systems, performance improvement, outcomes assessment and management, and growth of outpatient and partial treatment settings. All of these focus areas influence a facility's documentation requirements and will vary from organization to organization

Healthcare reform: A term used to refer to the concept of making changes to governmental policy that affects healthcare delivery within the United States. Generally, the emphasis of US healthcare reform is to improve the quality and safety of healthcare, improve access, and provide consumers with more choices at affordable prices while decreasing the overall costs of healthcare

Healthcare services: Processes that directly or indirectly contribute to the health and well-being of patients, such as medical, nursing, and other health-related services

Health Care and Education Reconciliation Act of 2010 (P.L. 111-152) (HCERA): A federal law enacted by Congress through reconciliation in order to make changes to the Patient Protection and Affordable Care Act. HCERA was signed into law by President Barack Obama on March 30, 2010; *Also called* HR 4872

Health Care Financing Administration (HCFA): Previous name of the Centers for Medicare and Medicaid Services

Health Care Provider Dimension (HCPD): One of three dimensions of the National Health Information

Infrastructure concept that includes information obtained during the patient care process and integrates it with clinical guidelines, protocols, and selected information the provider is authorized to access from the personal health record, as well as information relevant to the patient's care from the community health dimension

Health Care Quality Improvement Act (HCQIA): A 1986 act that requires facilities to report professional review actions on physicians, dentists, and other facility-based practitioners to the National Practitioner Data Bank (NPDB)

Health Care Quality Improvement Program (HCQIP): A quality initiative begun in 1992 by the Health Care Financing Administration and implemented by peer review organizations that uses patterns of care analysis and collaboration with practitioners, beneficiaries, providers, plans, and other purchasers of healthcare services to develop scientifically based quality indicators and to identify and implement opportunities for healthcare improvement

Health data: Includes both clinical and administrative data (and perhaps other data associated with an individual's healthcare); also includes aggregate-level health data for secondary uses, such as quality and patient safety monitoring, population health monitoring, research, and reimbursement

Health data analysis: The act of acquiring, collecting, evaluating, and processing health data by utilizing application skills such as database extraction and data analyzing tools to manage information contained in multiple large data sets

Health data analyst: Someone who uses application skills to manage, analyze, interpret, and transform health data into accurate, consistent, and timely information

Health data repository: A database that will provide immediate nationwide access to local data in the event of a primary system failure or system unavailability. It is an effort to improve data accessibility and increase disaster preparedness

Health delivery network: *See* **integrated provider organization**

Health Industry Business Communications Council (HIBCC): A subgroup of the American Standards

Committee X12 that focuses on electronic data interchange for billing transactions

Health informatics and information management (HIIM): Refers to the individuals responsible for managing healthcare data and information in paper or electronic form and controlling its collection, access, use, exchange, and protection through the application of health information technology

Health informatics standards: A set of standards that describe accepted methods for collecting, maintaining, and/or transferring healthcare data among computer systems

Health information: According to the HIPAA Privacy Rule, any information (verbal or written) created or received by a healthcare provider, health plan, public health authority, employer, life insurer, school or university, or healthcare clearinghouse that relates to the physical or mental health of an individual, provision of healthcare to an individual, or payment for provision of healthcare

Health information exchange (HIE): The exchange of health information electronically between providers and others with the same level of interoperability, such as labs and pharmacies

Health information exchange organization (HIEO): An organization that supports, oversees, or governs the exchange of health-related information among organizations according to nationally recognized standards

Health information management (HIM): An allied health profession that is responsible for ensuring the availability, accuracy, and protection of the clinical information that is needed to deliver healthcare services and to make appropriate healthcare-related decisions

Health Information Management and Systems Society (HIMSS): A national membership association that provides leadership in healthcare for the management of technology, information, and change

Health information management (HIM) department: Healthcare facility department responsible for the management and safeguarding of information in paper and electronic form

Health information management (HIM) professional: An individual who has received professional training at the associate or baccalaureate degree level in the management of health data and information flow throughout healthcare delivery systems; formerly known as **medical record technician** or **medical record administrator**

Health information management services (HIMS): One of several names for the health record department. This name is meant to provide a better description of the function of the department—the management of health information

Health Information National Trends Survey (HINTS): The National Cancer Institute's initiative that was to create a population-based survey that could be repeated biennially to track trends in the use of communication technology such as the Internet as a source of cancer information

Health information organization (HIO): An organization that supports, oversees, or governs the exchange of health-related information among organizations according to nationally recognized standards

Health information service provider (HSP): As described by the US HHS Office of the National Coordinator for Health Information Technology (ONC), a vendor that supplies the data integration and/or connectivity services for a health information organization

Health information services department: The department in a healthcare organization that is responsible for maintaining patient care records in accordance with external and internal rules and regulations; *Also called* **medical records department**

Health Information Standards Board (HISB): A subgroup of the American National Standards Institute that acts as an umbrella organization for groups interested in developing healthcare computer messaging standards

Health information technology (HIT): The technical aspects of processing health data and records, including classification and coding, abstracting, registry development, storage, and so on

Health Information Technology for Economic and Clinical Health Act (HITECH): Legislation created to stimulate the adoption of EHR and supporting technology in the United States. Signed into law on February 17, 2009, as part of ARRA.

Health information technology extension program: To assist healthcare providers to adopt, implement, and effectively use certified EHR technology that allows for the electronic exchange and use of health information, the Secretary, acting through the Office of the National Coordinator, shall establish a health information technology extension program to provide health information technology assistance services to be carried out through the Department of Health and Human Services. The National Coordinator shall consult with other federal agencies with demonstrated experience and expertise in information technology services, such as the National Institute of Standards and Technology, in developing and implementing this program

Health Information Technology Policy Committee: An HHS advisory committee that recommends the policy framework for the development and adoption of a nationwide health information infrastructure

Health Information Technology Regional Extension Center (HITREC or REC): Developed by the HITECH Act, these grants were designed to support and serve healthcare providers to help them quickly become adept and meaningful users of electronic health records (EHRs). RECs are designed to make sure that primary care clinicians get the help they need to use EHRs and provide training and support services to assist doctors and other providers in adopting EHRs

Health Information Technology Research Center (HITRC): Developed by the HITECH Act, this center is to gather information on effective practices and help the RECs work with one another and with relevant stakeholders to identify and share best practices in EHR adoption, meaningful use, and provider support

Health Information Technology Standards Committee: An HHS advisory committee that recommends standards, implementation specifications, and certification criteria for the electronic exchange and use of health information

Health Insurance Portability and Accountability Act of 1996 (HIPAA): The federal legislation enacted to provide continuity of health coverage, control fraud and abuse in healthcare, reduce healthcare costs, and guarantee the security and privacy of health information; limits exclusion for pre-existing medical conditions, prohibits discrimination against employees and dependents based on health status, guarantees availability of health insurance to small employers, and guarantees renewability of insurance to all employees regardless of size; requires covered entities (most healthcare providers and organizations) to transmit healthcare claims in a specific format and to develop, implement, and comply with the standards of the Privacy Rule and the Security Rule; and mandates that covered entities apply for and utilize national identifiers in HIPAA transactions; *Also called* the Kassebaum-Kennedy Law; **Public Law 104-191**

Health insurance prospective payment system (HIPPS) code: A five-character alphanumeric code used in the home health prospective payment system (HHPPS) and in the inpatient rehabilitation facility prospective payment system (IRFPPS). In the HHPPS, the HIPPS code is derived or computed from the home health resource group (HHRG); in the IRFPPS, the HIPPS code is derived from the case-mix group and comorbidity. Reimbursement weights for each HIPPS code correspond to the levels of care provided

Health insurance query for home health agencies (HIQH): An online transaction system that provides information on home health and hospice episodes for specific Medicare beneficiaries

Health Integrity and Protection Data Bank: A database maintained by the federal government to provide information on fraud-and-abuse findings against US healthcare providers

Health Level 7 (HL7): An international organization of healthcare professionals dedicated to creating standards for the exchange, management, and integration of electronic information

Health maintenance organization (HMO): Entity that combines the provision of healthcare insurance and the delivery of healthcare services, characterized by: (1) an organized healthcare delivery system to a geographic area, (2) a set of basic and supplemental health maintenance and treatment services, (3) voluntarily enrolled members, and (4) predetermined fixed, periodic prepayments for members' coverage

Health Maintenance Organization (HMO) Act: The 1973 federal legislation that outlined the requirements for federal qualifications of health maintenance organizations, consisting of legal and organizational structures, financial strength requirements, marketing provisions, and healthcare delivery

Health maintenance organization (HMO) referral: *See* **source of admission**

Health management information system (HMIS): An information system whose purpose is to provide reports on routine operations and processing (for example, a pharmacy inventory system, radiological system, or patient-tracking system)

Health plan: An entity that provides or pays the cost of medical care on behalf of enrolled individuals; includes group health plans, health insurance issuers, health maintenance organizations, and other welfare benefit plans such as Medicare, Medicaid, CHAMPUS, and Indian Health Services

Health Plan Employer Data and Information Set (HEDIS): A set of performance measures developed by the National Commission for Quality Assurance that are designed to provide purchasers and consumers of healthcare with the information they need to compare the performance of managed care plans

Health Privacy Project: A nonprofit organization whose mission is to raise public awareness of the importance of ensuring health privacy in order to improve healthcare access and quality

Health record: 1. Information relating to the physical or mental health or condition of an individual, as made by or on behalf of a health professional in connection with the care ascribed that individual 2. A medical record, health record, or medical chart that is a systematic documentation of a patient's medical history and care

Health record analysis: A concurrent or ongoing review of health record content performed by caregivers or HIM professionals while the patient is still receiving inpatient services to ensure the quality of the services being provided and the completeness of the documentation being maintained; *Also called* **health record review**

Health record banking: Health record banking is a new concept that is making headlines. This PHR model would allow patients and healthcare providers to share information by making deposits of health information into a bank. The health record bank would have to protect the privacy and security of the health information

Health record committee policy: A policy that outlines the goals of the committee, the audit tools used, the number of audits required and specific time frames for their completion, and the results-reporting mechanisms

Health record entry: The notation made in a patient's legal health record, whether paper or electronic, by the responsible healthcare practitioner to document an event or observation associated with healthcare services provided to the patient

Health record number: A unique numeric or alphanumeric identifier assigned to each patient's record upon admission to a healthcare facility

Health record ownership: The generally accepted principle that individual health records are maintained and owned by the healthcare organization that creates them but that patients have certain rights of control over the release of patient-identifiable (confidential) information

Health record review: *See* **health record analysis**

Health record security program: A set of processes and procedures designed to protect the data and information stored in a health record system from damage and unauthorized access

Health Research Extension Act (1985): Federal legislation that established guidelines for the proper care of animals used in biomedical and behavioral research

Health Resources and Services Administration (HRSA): The national organization that administers the State Children's Health Insurance Program along with the Centers for Medicare and Medicaid Services

Health savings accounts (HSAs): Savings accounts designed to help people save for future medical and retiree health costs on a tax-fee basis; part of the 2003 Medicare bill; *Also called* medical savings accounts

Health science librarian: A professional librarian who manages a medical library

Health services research: Research conducted on the subject of healthcare delivery that examines organizational structures and systems as well as the effectiveness and efficiency of healthcare services

Health systems agency (HSA): A type of organization called for by the Health Planning and Resources Development Act of 1974 to have broad representation of healthcare providers and consumers on governing boards and committees

Hearsay: A written or oral statement made outside of court that is offered in court as evidence

Hedge: A transaction that reduces the risk of an investment

HEDIS: *See* **Health Plan Employer Data and Information Set**

Help desk: A central access point to information system support services that attempts to resolve users' technical problems, sometimes with the use of decision-making algorithms, and tracks problems until their resolution

Helsinki Agreement: An ethical code established in 1964 by the 18th World Medical Assembly to guide researchers beyond the Nuremberg Code; differentiates between clinical or therapeutic research and nonclinical research and addresses problems with those who are legally incompetent and who need "proxy" representation

Hemodialysis: The process of removing metabolic waste products, toxins, and excess fluid from the bloodstream, accessed by an indwelling dialysis port

Heterogeneity: The state or fact of containing various components

Heuristic thought: Exploratory thinking that helps in solving certain types of problems but offers no guarantees

HFAP: *See* **Healthcare Facilities Accreditation Program**

HH: *See* **home health**

HHA: *See* **home health agency**

HHPPS: *See* **home health prospective payment system**

HHRG: *See* **home health resource group**

HHS: *See* **Department of Health and Human Services**

HIBCC: *See* **Health Industry Business Communications Council**

HIE: *See* **health information exchange**

Hierarchical system: A system structured with broad groupings that can be further subdivided into more narrowly defined groups or detailed entities

Hierarchy: An authoritarian organizational structure in which each member is assigned a specific rank that reflects his or her level of decision-making authority within the organization

Hierarchy of needs: Maslow's theory that suggested that human needs are organized hierarchically from basic physiological requirements to creative motivations; *See* **Maslow's Hierarchy of Needs**

High-cost outlier: *See* **outlier**

High-cost threshold: Criterion to assess whether technologies would be inadequately paid under the inpatient prospective payment system (IPPS): The sum of the geometric mean and the lesser of .75 of the national adjusted operating standardized payment amount (increased to reflect the difference between costs and charges) or .75 of one standard deviation of mean charges by diagnosis related group (DRG)

High-risk pool: An insurance plan (often a state healthcare insurance plan) that covers unhealthy or medically uninsurable people whose healthcare costs will be higher than average and whose utilization of healthcare services will be higher than average. Also the term for the small group of unhealthy individuals who have the high probability of incurring many healthcare services at high costs

Highly active antiretroviral therapy (HAART): A type of therapy that consists of multiple drugs commonly given to HIV-positive individuals before they develop AIDS

Highly sensitive health information: Certain types of patient information that require special handling in regard to access, requests, uses, and disclosures due to the nature of the information

HIIM: *See* **Health informatics and information management**

Hill-Burton Act: The federal legislation enacted in 1946 as the Hospital Survey and Construction Act to authorize grants for states to construct new hospitals and, later, to modernize old ones

HIM: *See* **health information management**

HIM professional: *See* **health information management professional**

HIMS: *See* **health information management services**

HIMSS: *See* **Healthcare Information and Management Systems Society**

HIPAA: *See* **Health Insurance Portability and Accountability Act of 1996**

HIPAA-grade encryption: Encrypted data or documents according to HIPAA Security and NIST 800-66 guidelines

HIPAA Privacy Rule: *See* **Health Insurance Portability and Accountability Act of 1996; Privacy Rule**

HIPAA Security Rule: *See* **Health Insurance Portability and Accountability Act of 1996; Security Rule**

HIPDB: *See* **Healthcare Integrity and Protection Data Bank**

Hippocratic oath: An oath created by ancient Greeks to embody a code of medical ethics

HIPPS code: *See* **health insurance prospective payment system code**

HIQH: *See* **health insurance query for home health agencies**

Hiring: Engaging the services of an individual in return for compensation

HIS: *See* **hospital information system**

HISB: *See* **Health Information Standards Board**

HISPC: *See* **Health Information Security and Privacy Collaboration**

Histocompatibility: The immunologic similarity between an organ donor and a transplant recipient

Histogram: A graphic technique used to display the frequency distribution of continuous data (interval or ratio data) as either numbers or percentages in a series of bars

Histology: The study of microscopic structure of tissue

Historical cost: The original resources expended by an organization to acquire an asset; considered the more objective measurement for financial reporting purposes

Historical-prospective study: Study design used when existing data sources can be used to identify characteristics pertaining to the study groups; groups followed over time, usually from the time data are first collected to the present or into the future, to examine their outcomes

Historical research: A research design used to investigate past events

History and physical (H&P): The pertinent information about the patient, including chief complaint, past and present illnesses, family history, social history, and review of body systems

History and physical documentation requirements policy: A policy that specifies the detail required in the history and physical examination done by the physician or physician extender

History of present illness (HPI): A chronological description of the development of the patient's present illness from the first sign and/or symptom or from the previous encounter to the present

History types: Generally defined by E/M services as: *problem-focused* (chief complaint; brief history of present illness or problem); *expanded problem-focused* (chief complaint; brief history of present illness; problem-pertinent system review); *detailed* (chief complaint; extended history of present illness; extended system review; pertinent past, family, and/or social history); and *comprehensive* (chief complaint; extended history of present illness; complete system review; complete past, family, and social history)

HIT: *See* **health information technology**

HITECH: *See* **Health Information Technology for Economic and Clinical Health Act**

HITRC: *See* **Health Information Technology Research Center**

HITREC: *See* **Health Information Technology Regional Extension Center**

HITSP: *See* **Healthcare Information Technology Standards Panel**

HIV: *See* **human immunodeficiency virus**

HL7: *See* **Health Level 7**

HL7 EHR Functional Model: A standard developed by HL7 that details the specifications for an electronic health record

HME: *See* **home medical equipment**

HMIS: *See* **health management information system**

HMO: *See* **health maintenance organization**

HMO Act: *See* **Health Maintenance Organization Act**

HMO referral: *See* **health maintenance organization referral**

HOLAP: *See* **hybrid online analytical processing**

Hold harmless: 1. Status in which one party does not hold the other party responsible 2. A term used to refer to the financial protections that ensure that cancer hospitals recoup all losses due to the differences in their ambulatory payment classification payments and the pre-APC payments for Medicare outpatient services

Home Assessment Validation and Entry (HAVEN): A type of data-entry software used to collect Outcome and Assessment Information Set (OASIS) data and then transmit them to state databases; imports and exports data in standard OASIS record format, maintains agency/patient/employee information, enforces data integrity through rigorous edit checks, and provides comprehensive online help. HAVEN is used in the home health prospective payment system (HHPPS)

Home care: *See* **home health**

Home health (HH): An umbrella term that refers to the medical and nonmedical services provided to patients and their families in their places of residence; *Also called* **home care**

Home health agency (HHA): A program or organization that provides a blend of home-based medical and social services to homebound patients and their families for the purpose of promoting, maintaining, or restoring health or of minimizing the effects of illness, injury, or disability; these services include skilled nursing care, physical therapy, occupational therapy, speech therapy, and personal care by home health aides

Home healthcare: The medical and/or personal care provided to individuals and families in their places of residence with the goal of promoting, maintaining, or restoring health or minimizing the effects of disabilities and illnesses, including terminal illnesses

Home health information system: An information system designed to support the care provided at a home health organization

Home health prospective payment system (HHPPS): The reimbursement system developed by the Centers for Medicare and Medicaid Services to cover home health services provided to Medicare beneficiaries

Home health resource group (HHRG): A classification system for the home health prospective payment system (HHPPS) derived from the data elements in the Outcome and Assessment Information Set (OASIS) with 80 home health episode rates established to support the prospective reimbursement of covered home care and rehabilitation services provided to Medicare beneficiaries during 60-day episodes of care; a six-character alphanumeric code is used to represent a severity level in three domains

Home medical equipment (HME): *See* **durable medical equipment**

Homeland Security Act: A 2002 act with the goal of preventing terrorist attacks in the United States while reducing the vulnerability of terrorism, minimizing its damages, and assisting in recovery from attacks in the United States. This act gives the government authorities the right to access health information needed to investigate and deter terrorism

Homogeneity: Variance in measurements or scores of the sample. Less variance, or greater homogeneity, in the measurements or scores of the sample results in narrower confidence intervals (CIs); greater variance and heterogeneity result in wider CIs

Honesty (integrity) tests: Tests designed to evaluate an individual's honesty using a series of hypothetical questions

HOPPS: *See* **Hospital Outpatient Prospective Payment System**

Horizontally integrated system: *See* **integrated provider organization**

Hospice: An interdisciplinary program of palliative care and supportive services that addresses the physical, spiritual, social, and economic needs of terminally ill patients and their families

Hospice care: The medical care provided to persons with life expectancies of six months or less who elect to forgo standard treatment of their illness and to receive only palliative care

Hospital: A healthcare entity that has an organized medical staff and permanent facilities that include inpatient beds and continuous medical or nursing services and that provides diagnostic and therapeutic services for patients as well as overnight accommodations and nutritional services

Hospital-acquired infection: An infection occurring in a patient in a hospital or healthcare setting in whom the infection was not present or incubating at the time of admission, or the remainder of an infection acquired during a previous admission; *See* **nosocomial infection**

Hospital-acquired infection rate: The number of hospital-acquired infections for a given time period divided by the total number of inpatient discharges for the same time period

Hospital-affiliated ambulatory surgery center: An ambulatory surgery center that is owned and operated by a hospital but is a separate entity with respect to its licensure, accreditation, governance, professional supervision, administrative functions, clinical services, record keeping, and financial and accounting systems

Hospital ambulatory care: All hospital-directed preventive, therapeutic, and rehabilitative services provided by physicians and their surrogates to patients who are not hospital inpatients

Hospital autopsy: A postmortem (after death) examination performed on the body of a person who has at some time been a hospital patient by a hospital pathologist or a physician of the medical staff who has been delegated the responsibility; *See* **hospital inpatient autopsy**

Hospital autopsy rate: The total number of autopsies performed by a hospital pathologist for a given time period divided by the number of deaths of hospital patients (inpatients and outpatients) whose bodies were available for autopsy for the same time period

Hospital autopsy rate, adjusted: The proportion of deaths of hospital patients following which the bodies were available for autopsy and hospital autopsies were performed; *See* **available for hospital autopsy**

Hospital-based ambulatory care center: An organized hospital facility that provides nonemergency medical or dental services to patients who are not assigned to a bed as inpatients during the time services are rendered (an emergency department in which services are provided to nonemergency patients is not considered an ambulatory care center)

Hospital-based ambulatory surgery center: A department of an inpatient facility that provides same-day surgical services using the facility's equipment, staff, and support services

Hospital-based eligible providers (EPs): An eligible provider such as a pathologist, anesthesiologist, or emergency physician, who furnishes substantially all of his or her Medicare-covered professional services during the relevant EHR reporting period in a hospital setting (whether inpatient or outpatient) through the use of the facilities and equipment of the hospital, including the hospital's qualified EHRs

Hospital-based outpatient care: A subset of ambulatory care that utilizes a hospital's staff, equipment, and resources to render preventive and/or corrective healthcare services

Hospital death rate: The number of inpatient deaths for a given period of time divided by the total number of live discharges and deaths for the same time period

Hospital discharge abstract system: A group of databases compiled from aggregate data on all patients discharged from a hospital

Hospital identification: A unique institutional number within a data collection system

Hospital (nosocomial) infection rate: The number of infections that occur in a hospital's various patient care units on a continuous basis

Hospital information system (HIS): The comprehensive database containing all the clinical, administrative, financial, and demographic information about each patient served by a hospital

Hospital inpatient: A patient who is provided with room, board, and continuous general nursing services in an area of an acute care facility where patients generally stay at least overnight

Hospital inpatient autopsy: A postmortem (after death) examination performed on the body of a patient who died during an inpatient hospitalization by a hospital pathologist or a physician of the medical staff who has been delegated the responsibility

Hospital inpatient beds: Accommodations with supporting services (such as food, laundry, and housekeeping) for hospital inpatients, excluding those for the newborn nursery but including incubators and bassinets in nurseries for premature or sick newborn infants

Hospital inpatient quality reporting program: Formerly known as the Reporting Hospital Quality Data for Annual Payment Update Program, this program is intended to equip consumers with quality of care information to make more informed decisions about healthcare options. Developed as a part of the Medicare Prescription Drug, Improvement and Modernization Act of 2003, it provided new requirements for quality reporting

Hospitalist: Physicians employed by teaching hospitals to play the role that admitting physicians fulfill in hospitals that are not affiliated with medical training programs

Hospitalization: The period during an individual's life when he or she is a patient in a single hospital without interruption except by possible intervening leaves of absence; *See* **inpatient hospitalization**

Hospitalization insurance (Medicare Part A): A federal program that covers the costs associated with inpatient hospitalization as well as other healthcare services provided to Medicare beneficiaries

Hospital live birth: In an inpatient facility, the complete expulsion or extraction of a product of human conception from the mother, regardless of the duration of pregnancy, which, after such expulsion or extraction, breathes or shows any other evidence of life, such as beating of the heart, pulsation of the umbilical cord, or definite movement of voluntary muscles

Hospital newborn bassinet: Accommodations including incubators and isolettes in the newborn nursery with supporting services (such as food, laundry, and housekeeping) for hospital newborn inpatients

Hospital newborn inpatient: A patient born in the hospital at the beginning of the current inpatient hospitalization

Hospital outpatient: A hospital patient who receives services in one or more of a hospital's facilities when he or she is not currently an inpatient or a home care patient

Hospital outpatient care unit: An organized unit of a hospital that provides facilities and medical services exclusively or primarily to patients who are generally ambulatory and who do not currently require or are not currently receiving services as an inpatient of the hospital

Hospital Outpatient Prospective Payment System (HOPPS): The reimbursement system created by the Balanced Budget Act of 1997 for hospital outpatient services rendered to Medicare beneficiaries; maintained by the Centers for Medicare and Medicaid Services (CMS)

Hospital outpatient Quality Data Reporting Program (HOP QDRP): Quality-based pay-for-performance program implemented for HOPPS facilities in CY 2009.

Hospitals must report data for measures established by CMS in order to receive a full HOPPS rate update

Hospital Payment Monitoring Program (HPMP): Coding compliance monitoring program created by the 7th Scope of Work which ensures that proper payment is made for Medicare beneficiary admissions

Hospital Standardization Program: An early 20th-century survey mechanism instituted by the American College of Surgeons and aimed at identifying quality-of-care problems and improving patient care; precursor to the survey program offered by the Joint Commission

Hospital within hospital (HwH): Long-term care hospital physically located within another hospital

Hot site: A duplicate of the organization's critical systems stored in a remote location

House of Delegates: An important component of the volunteer structure of the American Health Information Management Association that conducts the official business of the organization and functions as its legislative body

House staff: A physician in training who is continuing his or her medical education in a residency program, working with specialists to obtain higher-level skills and experience treating patients

H&P: *See* **history and physical**

HPD: *See* **healthcare provider dimension**

HPI: *See* **history of present illness**

HPMP: *See* **Hospital Payment Monitoring Program**

HPSA: Health professional shortage area

HRSA: *See* **Health Resources and Services Administration**

HSA: *See* **health systems agency**

HSAs: *See* **health savings accounts**

HTML: *See* **hypertext markup language**

HTTP: *See* **hypertext transport protocol**

HUGN: *See* **Human Genome Nomenclature**

Human–computer interface: The device used by humans to access and enter data into a computer system, such as a keyboard on a PC, personal digital assistant, voice recognition system, and so on

Human Genome Nomenclature (HUGN): Interoperability standard for exchanging information regarding the role of genes in biomedical research and healthcare

Human Genome Project: A multiyear project ending in 2003 which involved the identification and mapping of all human DNA

Human immunodeficiency virus (HIV): The virus that causes acquired immunodeficiency syndrome (AIDS)

Human relations movement: A management philosophy emphasizing the shift from a mechanistic view of workers to concern for their satisfaction at work

Human resources: The employees of an organization

Human subjects: Individuals whose physiologic or behavioral characteristics and responses are the object of study in a research program

Human systems: Systems that are organized relationships among people

Hybrid entity: An entity that performs both covered and noncovered functions under the Privacy Rule; for example, a university that educates students and maintains student educational records is not covered by the Privacy Rule; however, the same university that operates a medical center is covered by the Privacy Rule as it meets the definition of "healthcare provider"

Hybrid health record: A combination of paper and electronic records; a health record that includes both paper and electronic elements

Hybrid online analytical processing (HOLAP): A data access methodology that is coupled tightly with the architecture of the database management system to allow the user to perform business analyses

Hypertext markup language (HTML): A standardized computer language that allows the electronic transfer of information and communications among many different information systems

Hypertext transport protocol (HTTP): A communications protocol that enables the use of hypertext linking

Hyperthermia: The use of heat to raise the temperature of a specific area of the body in an attempt to increase cell metabolism

Hypothesis: A statement that describes a research question in measurable terms

Iatrogenic: Induced inadvertently by a physician or surgeon or by medical treatment or diagnostic procedures

ICCE: Intracapsular cataract extraction

ICD-9-CM: A classification system used in the United States to report morbidity and mortality information; *See* **International Classification of Diseases, ninth revision, Clinical Modification**

ICD-9-CM Coordination and Maintenance Committee: Committee composed of representatives from the National Center for Health Statistics (NCHS) and the Centers for Medicare and Medicaid Services (CMS) that is responsible for maintaining the United States' clinical modification version of the International Classification of Diseases, ninth revision (ICD-9-CM) code sets; holds open meetings that serve as a public forum for discussing (but not making decisions about) proposed revisions to ICD-9-CM

ICD-O-3: *See* **International Classification of Diseases for Oncology, Third Edition**

ICD-10: *See* **International Classification of Diseases, tenth revision**

ICD-10-CM: *See* **International Classification of Diseases, tenth revision, Clinical Modification**

ICD-10-PCS: *See* **International Classification of Diseases, tenth revision, Procedure Coding System**

ICF: *See* **intermediate care facility; International Classification on Functioning, Disability and Health**

ICH: *See* **International Conference on Harmonization of Technical Requirements for Registration of Pharmaceuticals for Human Use**

ICN: *See* **International Council of Nurses**

ICNP: *See* **International Classification for Nursing Practice**

ICNP Catalogues: A set of precoordinated statements being developed by the International Council of Nurses that will consist of subsets of nursing diagnoses, interventions, and outcomes for a specific area of practice

Icon: A graphic symbol used to represent a critical event in a process flowchart

ICPC-2: *See* **International Classification of Primary Care**

ICU: Intensive care unit

Identifier standards: Recommended methods for assigning unique identifiers to individuals (patients and clinical providers), corporate providers, and healthcare vendors and suppliers

Identity management: In the master patient index, policies and procedures that manage patient identity, such as prohibiting the same record number for duplicate patients or duplicate records for one patient

IDR technology: *See* **intelligent document recognition technology**

IDS: *See* **integrated delivery system**

IEEE: *See* **Institute of Electrical and Electronics Engineers**

IETF: *See* **Internet Engineering Task Force**

IFA: *See* **indirect immunofluorescence assay**

IGC: *See* **impairment group code**

IHI: *See* **Institute for Healthcare Improvement**

IHS: *See* **Indian Health Service**

Image processing: The ability of a computer to create a graphic representation of a text block, photograph, drawing, or other image and make it available throughout an information system

Imaging technology: Computer software designed to combine health record text files with diagnostic imaging files

IME adjustment: *See* **indirect medical education adjustment**

Immunoassay: Detection and evaluation of substances by serological (immunologic) methods

Impact analysis: A collective term used to refer to any study that determines the benefit of a proposed project, including cost-benefit analysis, return on investment, benefits realization study, or qualitative benefit study

Impairment group code (IGC): Multidigit code that represents the primary reason for a patient's admission to an inpatient rehabilitation facility

Impairment rider: *See* **exclusion**

Implementation phase: The third phase of the systems development life cycle during which a comprehensive plan is developed and instituted to ensure that the new information system is effectively implemented within the organization

Implementation specifications: Descriptions that define how HIPAA standards are to be implemented

Implied consent: The type of permission that is inferred when a patient voluntarily submits to treatment

Incentive: Something that stimulates or encourages an individual to work harder

Incentive pay: A system of bonuses and rewards based on employee productivity; often used in transcription areas of healthcare facilities

Incidence: The number of new cases of a specific disease

Incidence rate: A computation that compares the number of new cases of a specific disease for a given time period to the population at risk for the disease during the same time period

Incident: An occurrence in a medical facility that is inconsistent with accepted standards of care

Incident report: A quality or performance management tool used to collect data and information about potentially compensable events (events that may result in death or serious injury); *See also* **occurrence report**

Incident report review: An analysis of incident reports or an evaluation of descriptions of adverse events

Incisional breast biopsy: A type of breast biopsy done through an incision that does not include removal of the entire lesion

Income statement: A statement that summarizes an organization's revenue and expense accounts using totals accumulated during the fiscal year

Incomplete records policy: A policy that outlines how physicians are notified of records missing documentation and/or signatures

Incremental budgeting: A budgeting approach in which the financial database of the past is increased by a given percentage and adjustments are made for anticipated changes, with an added inflation factor

Indemnification statement: A statement that exempts the signer from incurring liabilities or penalties

Indemnity health insurance: Traditional, fee-for-service healthcare plan in which the policyholder pays a monthly premium and a percentage of the usual, customary, and reasonable healthcare costs and the patient can select the provider

Indemnity plans: Health insurance coverage provided in the form of cash payments to patients or providers; *See* **indemnity health insurance**

Independent consultant: An individual who works as a contractor to provide HIM services to healthcare facilities

Independent practice organization (IPO) or association (IPA): An open-panel health maintenance organization that provides contract healthcare services to subscribers through independent physicians who treat patients in their own offices; the HMO reimburses the IPA on a capitated basis; the IPA may reimburse the physicians on a fee-for-service or a capitated basis; *Also called* **foundation model**; **individual practice association model**

Independent practitioners: Individuals working as employees of an organization, in private practice, or through a physician group who provide healthcare services without supervision or direction

Independent variables: The factors in experimental research that researchers manipulate directly

Index: An organized (usually alphabetical) list of specific data that serves to guide, indicate, or otherwise facilitate reference to the data

Indian Health Service (IHS): The federal agency within the Department of Health and Human Services that is responsible for providing federal healthcare services to American Indians and Alaska natives

Indicator: An activity, event, occurrence, or outcome that is to be monitored and evaluated under the Joint Commission standard in order to determine whether those aspects conform to standards; commonly relates to the structure, process, and/or outcome of an important aspect of care; *Also called* a **criterion** 2. A measure used to determine an organization's performance over time

Indicator measurement system: An indicator-based monitoring system developed by the Joint Commission for accredited organizations and meant to provide hospitals with information on their performance

Indirect costs: Resources expended that cannot be identified as pertaining to specific goods and/or services (for example, electricity is not allocable to a specific patient)

Indirect immunofluorescence assay (IFA): One of the diagnostic tests used to confirm infection with the human immunodeficiency virus (HIV)

Indirect laryngoscopy: A procedure that enables the larynx to be viewed with a laryngeal mirror

Indirect medical education (IME) adjustment: Percentage increase in Medicare reimbursement to offset the costs of medical education that a teaching hospital incurs

Indirect obstetric death: The death of a woman that resulted from a previously existing disease (or a disease that developed during pregnancy, labor, or the puerperium) that was not due to obstetric causes, although the physiologic effects of pregnancy were partially responsible for the death

Individual: According to the HIPAA Privacy Rule, a person who is the subject of protected health information

Individually identifiable health information: According to HIPAA privacy provisions, that information which specifically identifies the patient to whom the information relates, such as age, gender, date of birth, and address

Individual practice association model: *See* **independent practice organization**

Individual provider: A health professional who delivers or is professionally responsible for delivering services to a patient, is exercising independent judgment in the care of the patient, and is not under the immediate supervision of another healthcare professional

Induced termination of pregnancy: The purposeful interruption of an intrauterine pregnancy that did not result in a live birth

Inductive reasoning: A process of creating conclusions based on a limited number of observations

Industry standard: The procedures and/or criteria that have been recognized as acceptable practices by peer professional, credentialing, and/or accrediting organizations

Infant death: The death of a live-born infant at any time from the moment of birth to the end of the first year of life (364 days, 23 hours, 59 minutes from the moment of birth)

Infant mortality rate: The number of deaths of individuals under one year of age during a given time period divided by the number of live births reported for the same time period

Infection control: A system for the prevention of communicable diseases that concentrates on protecting healthcare workers and patients against exposure to disease-causing organisms and promotes compliance with applicable legal requirements through early identification of potential sources of contamination and implementation of policies and procedures that limit the spread of disease

Infection rate: The ratio of all infections to the number of discharges, including deaths

Infection review: Evaluation of the risk of infection among patients and healthcare providers, looking for, preventing, and controlling the risk

Inference engine: Specialized computer software that tries to match conditions in rules to data elements in a repository (when a match is found, the engine executes the rule, which results in the occurrence of a specified action)

Inferential statistics: 1. Statistics that are used to make inferences from a smaller group of data to a large one 2. A set of statistical techniques that allows researchers to make generalizations about a population's characteristics (parameters) on the basis of a sample's characteristics

Informaticians: Individuals in a field of study (informatics) that focuses on the use of technology to improve access to, and utilization of, information

Informatics: A field of study that focuses on the use of technology to improve access to, and utilization of, information

Information: Data that have been deliberately selected, processed, and organized to be useful

Information assets: Information that has value for an organization

Information capture: The process of recording representations of human thought, perceptions, or actions in documenting patient care, as well as device-generated information that is gathered and/or computed about a patient as part of healthcare

Information integrity: The dependability or trustworthiness of information. It concerns more than data quality or data accuracy—it encompasses the entire framework in which information is recorded, processed, and used

Information kiosk: A computer station located within a healthcare facility that patients and families can use to access information

Information life cycle: The cycle of gathering, recording, processing, storing, sharing, transmitting, retrieving, and deleting information

Information management: The generation, collection, organization, validation, analysis, storage, and integration of data as well as the dissemination, communication, presentation, utilization, transmission, and safeguarding of the information

Information model: A model that combines the elements necessary to fully represent the meaning of clinical information and that supports semantic interoperability among the heterogeneous computer-based systems that form an integrated information system

Information modeling: The use of clinical code sets with application software to create information that is meaningful to the end user

Information resource management: A concept that assumes that information is a valuable resource that must be managed, regardless of the form it takes or the medium in which it is stored

Information science: The study of the nature and principles of information

Information security program: A program that includes all activities of an organization related to information security, including policies, standards, training, technical and procedural controls, risk assessment, auditing and monitoring, and assigned responsibility for management of the program

Information services department: *See* **health information services department**

Information system (IS): An automated system that uses computer hardware and software to record, manipulate, store, recover, and disseminate data (that is, a system that receives and processes input and provides output); often used interchangeably with **information technology (IT)**

Information systems (IS) department: The department in a healthcare organization that is responsible for ensuring that the organization has the technical infrastructure and staff required to operate and manage its computer-based systems

Information technology (IT): 1. Computer technology (hardware and software) combined with telecommunications technology (data, image, and voice networks); often used interchangeably with **information system (IS)** 2. A term that encompasses most forms of technology used to create, store, exchange, and use electronic information

Information technology (IT) professional: An individual who works with computer technology in the process of managing health information

Information technology (IT) strategy: An organization's information technology goals, objectives, and strategic plans, which serve as a guide to the procurement of information systems within an organization

Informed consent: 1. A legal term referring to a patient's right to make his or her own treatment decisions based on the knowledge of the treatment to be administered or the procedure to be performed 2. An individual's voluntary agreement to participate in research or to undergo a diagnostic, therapeutic, or preventive medical procedure

Infrastructure: The underlying framework and features of an information system

Initiating structure: Leaders in this group were more task-focused and centered on giving direction, setting goals and limits, and planning and scheduling activities

Injury (harm): In a negligence lawsuit, one of four elements, which may be economic (hospital expenses and loss of wages) and noneconomic (pain and suffering), that must be proved to be successful

Injury Severity Score (ISS): An overall severity measurement maintained in the trauma registry and calculated from the abbreviated injury scores for the three most severe injuries of each patient

Innovator: An early adopter of change who is eager to experiment with new ways of doing things

Inpatient: *See* **hospital inpatient**

Inpatient admission: An acute care facility's formal acceptance of a patient who is to be provided with room, board, and continuous nursing service in an area of the facility where patients generally stay at least overnight

Inpatient bed count: *See* **bed count**

Inpatient bed occupancy rate: The total number of inpatient service days for a given time period divided by the total number of inpatient bed count days for the same time period; *Also called* **percentage of occupancy**

Inpatient census: *See* census

Inpatient coding compliance: The accurate and complete assignment of ICD-9-CM diagnostic and procedural codes, along with appropriate sequencing (for example, identification of principal diagnosis) to determine the appropriate diagnosis-related group and resultant payment

Inpatient daily census: The number of inpatients present at census-taking time each day, plus any inpatients who were both admitted and discharged after the previous day's census-taking time

Inpatient days of stay: *See* **length of stay**

Inpatient discharge: The termination of hospitalization through the formal release of an inpatient from a hospital; *See also* **discharge status**

Inpatient hospitalization: The period during an individual's life when he or she is a patient in a single hospital without interruption except by possible intervening leaves of absence

Inpatient long-term care hospital (LTCH): A healthcare facility that has an average length of stay greater than 25 days, with patients classified into distinct diagnosis groups called MS-LTC-DRGs; prospective payment system for LTCHs was established by CMS and went into effect beginning in 2002

Inpatient psychiatric facility (IPF): A healthcare facility that offers psychiatric medical care on an inpatient basis

Inpatient psychiatric facility PPS (IPFPPS): A per diem prospective payment system that is based on 15 diagnosis-related groups, which became effective on January 1, 2005

Inpatient rehabilitation facility (IRF): A healthcare facility that specializes in providing services to patients who have suffered a disabling illness or injury in an effort to help them achieve or maintain their optimal level of functioning, self-care, and independence

Inpatient rehabilitation facility PPS (IRFPPS): Utilizes the patient assessment instrument to assign patients to case-mix groups according to their clinical situation and resource requirements

Inpatient Rehabilitation Validation and Entry (IRVEN): A computerized data-entry system used by inpatient rehabilitation facilities (IRFs). Captures data for the IRF Patient Assessment Instrument (IRF PAI) and supports electronic submission of the IRF PAI. Also allows data import and export in the standard record format of the Centers for Medicare and Medicaid Services (CMS)

Inpatient service day (IPSD): A unit of measure equivalent to the services received by one inpatient during one 24-hour period

Inputs: Data entered into a hospital system (for example, the patient's knowledge of his or her condition, the admitting clerk's knowledge of the admission process, and the computer with its admitting template are all inputs for the hospital's admitting system)

Insertion: Putting in a nonbiological device that monitors, assists, performs, or prevents a physiological function but does not physically take the place of the body part

In-service education: Training that teaches employees specific skills required to maintain or improve performance, usually internal to an organization

Inspection: Visually and/or manually exploring a body part. May be performed with or without optical instrumentation. May be performed directly or through intervening body layers

Install base: The number of clients for which a vendor has installed a system, as opposed to the number of clients for which a vendor is in the process of selling a system

Institute for Clinical Systems Improvement (ICSI): A collaboration of healthcare organizations that provides an objective voice dedicated to supporting healthcare quality and helping its members identify and achieve implementation of best practices for their patients

Institute of Electrical and Electronics Engineers (IEEE): A national organization that develops standards for hospital system interface transactions, including links between critical care bedside instruments and clinical information systems

Institute of Electrical and Electronics Engineers Standards Association (IEEE-SA): An activity of the IEEE that develops standards in a broad range of industries including healthcare

Institute of Electrical and Electronics Engineers (IEEE) 1073: Interoperability standard for electronic data exchange

Institute for Healthcare Improvement (IHI): A quality and safety improvement group partnering with patients and healthcare professionals to promote safe and effective healthcare

Institute of Medicine (IOM): A branch of the National Academy of Sciences whose goal is to advance and distribute scientific knowledge with the mission of improving human health

Institutional death rate: *See* **net death rate**

Institutional Review Board (IRB): An administrative body that provides review, oversight, guidance, and approval for research projects carried out by employees serving as researchers, regardless of the location of the research (such as a university or private research agency); responsible for protecting the rights and welfare of the human subjects involved in the research. IRB oversight is mandatory for federally funded research projects

Instrument: A standardized and uniform way to measure and collect data

Insurance: 1. A purchased contract (policy) according to which the purchaser (insured) is protected from loss by the insurer's agreeing to reimburse for such loss 2. Reduction of a person's (insured's) exposure to risk by having another party (insurer) assume the risk

Insurance certification: The process of determining that the patient has insurance coverage for the treatment that is planned or expected

Insurance code mapping: The methodology that allows a hospital to hold more than one CPT/HCPCS code per chargemaster item

Insured: A holder of a health insurance policy; *See* **certificate holder**; **member**; **policyholder**; **subscriber**

Insurer: An organization that pays healthcare expenses on behalf of its enrollees; *See* **third-party payer**

Integrated delivery network (IDN): *See* **integrated delivery system**

Integrated delivery system (IDS): A system that combines the financial and clinical aspects of healthcare and uses a group of healthcare providers, selected on the basis of quality and cost management criteria, to furnish comprehensive health services across the continuum of care; *See* **integrated provider organization**

Integrated healthcare network: A group of healthcare organizations that collectively provides a full range of coordinated healthcare services ranging from simple preventative care to complex surgical care

Integrated health record format: A system of health record organization in which all the paper forms are arranged in strict chronological order and mixed with forms created by different departments

Integrated health records: *See* **integrated health record format**

Integrated health system: *See* **integrated delivery system**

Integrated provider organization (IPO): An organization that manages the delivery of healthcare services provided by hospitals, physicians (employees of the IPO), and other healthcare organizations (for example, nursing facilities); *See* **integrated delivery system**

Integrated service network (ISN): *See* **integrated provider organization (IPO)**

Integrated services digital network (ISDN): A computer system that transmits voice, data, and signaling digitally and with significantly increased bandwidth compared to traditional T-1 lines

Integration: The complex task of ensuring that all elements and platforms in an information system communicate and act as a uniform entity; or the combination of two or more benefit plans to prevent duplication of benefit payment

Integration testing: A form of testing during EHR implementation performed to ensure that the interfaces between applications and systems work

Integrative review: *See* **systematic literature review**

Integrity: 1. The state of being whole or unimpaired 2. The ability of data to maintain its structure and attributes, including protection against modification or corruption during transmission, storage, or at rest. Maintenance of data integrity is a key aspect of data quality management and security

Integrity constraints: Limits placed on the data that may be entered into a database

Intellectual capital: The combined knowledge of an organization's employees with respect to operations, processes, history, and culture

Intellectual property: A legal term that refers to creative thoughts that, when they generate a unique solution to a problem, may take on value and thus can become a commodity

Intelligent character recognition (ICR) technology: A method of encoding handwritten, print, or cursive characters and of interpreting the characters as words or the intent of the writer; *See* **gesture recognition technology**

Intelligent document recognition (IDR) technology: A form of technology that automatically recognizes analog items, such as tangible materials or documents, or recognizes characters or symbols from analog items, enabling the identified data to be quickly, accurately, and automatically entered into digital systems

Intelligent prompting: A means in tables and forms for displaying only clinically relevant items

Intensity of service (IS or IOS): A type of supportive documentation that reflects the diagnostic and therapeutic services for a specified level of care

Intensity-of-service (IS) screening criteria: Preestablished standards used to determine the most efficient healthcare setting in which to safely provide needed services

Intensive review: A process undertaken when an incident occurs that requires the review of medical record or other data elements to determine if process problems exist and if an ongoing performance measure should be established to monitor process stability

Intentional tort: A circumstance where a healthcare provider purposely commits a wrongful act that results in injury

Interactive voice response: An automated call handler that can be configured to automatically dial a log of callers and deliver appointment reminders, lab results, and other information when a person answers the phone

Interactive voice technology (IVT): A communications technology that enables an individual to use a telephone to access information from a computer

Interagency transfer form: A form that contains sufficient information about a patient to provide continuity of care during transfer or discharge

Interest: The cost of borrowing money; payment to creditors for using money on credit

Interface: The zone between different computer systems across which users want to pass information (for example, a computer program written to exchange information between systems or the graphic display of an application program designed to make the program easier to use)

Interface management: The identification, definition, and control of interfaces to ensure that the system operates as expected

Interim payment system (IPS): A cost-based reimbursement system that was used until the prospective payment system was phased in

Interim period: Any period that represents less than an entire fiscal year

Intermediate care facility: A facility that provides health-related care and services to individuals who do not require the degree of care or treatment that a hospital or a skilled nursing facility provides but who still require medical care and services because of their physical or mental condition

Intermediate fetal death: The death of a product of human conception before its complete expulsion or extraction from the mother that is 20 complete weeks of gestation (but less than 28 weeks) and weighs 501 to 1,000 grams

Internal controls: Policies and procedures designed to protect an organization's assets and to reduce the exposure to the risk of loss due to error or malfeasance

Internal data: Data from within the facility that include administrative and clinical data

Internal rate of return (IRR): An interest rate that makes the net present value calculation equal zero

Internal validity: An attribute of a study's design that contributes to the accuracy of its findings

International Classification for Nursing Practice (ICNP): Unified nursing language system into which existing terminologies can be cross-mapped

International Classification of Diseases for Oncology, Third Edition (ICD-O-3): A system used for classifying incidences of malignant disease

International Classification of Diseases, Ninth Revision, Clinical Modification (ICD-9-CM): A coding and classification system used in the United States to report diagnoses in all healthcare settings and inpatient procedures and services as well as morbidity and mortality information

International Classification of Diseases, Tenth Revision (ICD-10): The most recent revision of the disease classification system developed and used by the World Health Organization to track morbidity and mortality information worldwide (not yet adopted by the United States)

International Classification of Diseases, Tenth Revision, Clinical Modification (ICD-10-CM): The coding classification system that will replace ICD-9-CM, Volumes 1 and 2, on October 1, 2013. ICD-10-CM is the United States' clinical modification of the World Health Organization's ICD-10. ICD-10-CM has a total of 21 chapters and contains significantly more codes than ICD-9-CM, providing the ability to code with a greater level of specificity

International Classification of Diseases, Tenth Revision, Procedure Coding System (ICD-10-PCS): The coding classification system that will replace ICD-9-CM, Volume 3, on October 1, 2013. ICD-10-PCS has 16 sections and contains significantly more procedure codes than ICD-9-CM, providing the ability to code procedures with a greater level of specificity

International Classification of Impairments, Disabilities, and Handicaps (ICIDH): Published by the World Health Organization to measure the consequences of disease and divided into three classifications: impairments, disabilities, and handicaps; the precursor to ICF

International Classification of Primary Care (ICPC-2): Classification used for coding the reasons of encounter, diagnoses, and interventions in an episode-of-care structure

International Classification on Functioning, Disability and Health (ICF): Classification of health and health-related domains that describe body functions and structures, activities, and participation

International Conference on Harmonization of Technical Requirements for Registration of Pharmaceuticals for Human Use (ICH): A joint project established in 1990 that brings together the drug regulatory authorities of the European Union (European Medicines Evaluation Agency), Japan (Ministry of Health and Welfare), and the United States (Food and Drug Administration) as well as representative associations of the pharmaceutical research-based industry in the three regions

International Council of Nurses (ICN): A federation of national nurses' associations representing millions of nurses worldwide that was instrumental in developing the International Classification for Nursing Practice

International Federation of Health Record Organizations (IFHRO): Organization that supports national associations and health record professionals to implement and improve health records and the systems that support them

International Health Terminology Standards Development Organization: A company based in Denmark that is responsible for maintaining SNOMED International, a method for encoding data variables when physicians enter data into a history and physical exam template

International Medical Informatics Association (IMIA): Worldwide not-for-profit organization that promotes medical informatics in healthcare and biomedical research

International Organization for Standardization (ISO): The world's largest developer of standards whose principal activity is the development of technical standards, which often have important economic and social repercussions

Internet: An international network of computer servers that provides individual users with communications channels and access to software and information repositories worldwide

Internet browsers: A type of client software that facilitates communications among World Wide Web information servers

Internet Engineering Task Force (IETF): A group that reviews and issues Internet standards

Internet protocol (IP) telephony: A type of communications technology that allows people to initiate real-time calls through the Internet instead of the public telephone system; *See* **voiceover IP (VoIP)**

Internet service provider (ISP): A company that provides connections to the Internet

Interoperability: The ability of different information systems and software applications to communicate and exchange data

Interpersonal skills: One of the three managerial skill categories that includes skills in communicating and relating effectively to others

Interpreter: A type of communications technology that converts high-level language statements into machine language one at a time

Interrater reliability: A measure of a research instrument's consistency in data collection when used by different abstractors

Interrogatories: Discovery devices consisting of a set of written questions given to a party, witness, or other person who has information needed in a legal case

Interrupted stay case: 1. A rehabilitation stay interrupted by a single admission to an acute care hospital 2. Discharge in which the patient was discharged from the inpatient rehabilitation facility and returned within three calendar days

Interval data: A type of data that represents observations that can be measured on an evenly distributed scale beginning at a point other than true zero

Interval-level data: Data with a defined unit of measure, no true zero point, and equal intervals between successive values; *See* **ratio-level data**

Interval note: Health record documentation that describes the patient's course between two closely related hospitalizations directed toward the treatment of the same complaint when a patient has been discharged and readmitted within 30 days

Interval scale: Situation where the intervals between adjacent scale values are equal with respect to the attributes being measured

Intervention: 1. A clinical manipulation, treatment, or therapy 2. A generic term used by researchers to mean an act of some kind

Interventional radiology: The branch of medicine that diagnoses and treats a wide range of diseases using percutaneous or minimally invasive techniques under imaging guidance

Interview: A formal meeting, often between a job applicant and a potential employer

Interview guide: A list of written questions to be asked during an interview

Interview survey: A type of research instrument with which the members of the population being studied are asked questions and respond orally

Intracapsular lens extraction: The surgical removal of the entire lens and its capsule, generally followed by insertion of an anterior chamber intraocular lens

Intrahospital transfer: A change in medical care unit, medical staff unit, or responsible physician during hospitalization

Intranet: A private information network that is similar to the Internet and whose servers are located inside a firewall or security barrier so that the general public cannot gain access to information housed within the network

Intraoperative anesthesia record: Health record documentation that describes the entire surgical process from the time the operation began until the patient left the operating room

Intrarater reliability: A measure of a research instrument's reliability in which the same person repeating the test will get reasonably similar findings

Intuition: Unconscious decision making based on extensive experience in similar situations

Inventor: A role in organizational innovation that requires idea generation

Inventory: Goods on hand and available to sell, presumably within a year (a business cycle)

Inventory control: The balance between purchasing and storing the supplies needed and not wasting money or space should the requirements for that supply change or the space available for storage be limited

Inverse relationship: *See* **negative relationship**

Investor-owned hospital chain: Group of for-profit healthcare facilities owned by stockholders

IOL: Intraocular lens

IOM: *See* **Institute of Medicine**

IOS: *See* **intensity of service**

IPA: *See* **independent practice association**

IPF: *See* **inpatient psychiatric facility**

IPFPPS: *See* **inpatient psychiatric facility PPS**

IPO: *See* **independent practice organization; integrated provider organization**

IPPB: intermittent positive pressure breathing

IPS: *See* **interim payment system**

Ipsilateral: Situated or appearing on the same side, or affecting the same side of the body

IP telephony: *See* **Internet protocol telephony**

IRB: *See* **institutional review board**

IRF: *See* **inpatient rehabilitation facility**

IRF PAI: *See* **inpatient rehabilitation facility patient assessment instrument**

IRFPPS: *See* **inpatient rehabilitation facility PPS**

IRR: *See* **internal rate of return**

IRVEN: *See* **Inpatient Rehabilitation Validation and Entry**

IS: *See* **information system; intensity of service**

IS-A relationships: Parent-child relationships that link concepts within a hierarchy

IS department: *See* **information systems department**

ISDN: *See* **integrated services digital network**

ISN: *See* **integrated service network**

ISO: *See* **International Organization for Standardization; United Nations International Standards Organization**

ISO 9000: An internationally agreed-upon set of generic standards for quality management systems established by the International Standards Organization

ISP: *See* **Internet service provider**

ISS: *See* **injury severity score**

IS/SI criteria: *See* **intensity-of-service screening criteria; severity-of-illness screening criteria**

Issue log: A form of documentation that describes the questions, concerns, and problems that must be solved in order for a task to be completed

Issues management: The process of identifying causes, resolving unexpected occurrences, and maintaining a level of problem or error control

IT: *See* **information technology**

Item description: An explanation of a service or supply listed in the chargemaster

IT professional: *See* **information technology professional**

IT strategy: *See* **information technology strategy**

IV: intravenous

IVT: *See* **interactive voice technology**

JIT: *See* **just-in-time training**

Job classification method: 1. A method of job evaluation that compares a written position description with the written descriptions of various classification grades 2. A method used by the federal government to grade jobs

Job description: A detailed list of a job's duties, reporting relationships, working conditions, and responsibilities; *See* **position description**

Job evaluation: The process of applying predefined compensable factors to jobs to determine their relative worth

Job procedure: A structured, action-oriented list of sequential steps involved in carrying out a specific task or solving a problem

Job ranking: A method of job evaluation that arranges jobs in a hierarchy on the basis of each job's importance to the organization, with the most important jobs listed at the top of the hierarchy and the least important jobs listed at the bottom

Job redesign: The process of realigning the needs of the organization with the skills and interests of the employee and then designing the job to meet those needs (for example, in order to introduce new tools or technology or provide better customer service)

Job rotation: A work design in which workers are shifted periodically among different tasks

Job sharing: A work schedule in which two or more individuals share the tasks of one full-time or one full-time-equivalent position

Job specifications: A list of a job's required education, skills, knowledge, abilities, personal qualifications, and physical requirements

The Joint Commission: A private, voluntary, not-for-profit organization that evaluates and accredits hospitals and other healthcare organizations on the basis of predefined performance standards; formerly known as the Joint Commission on Accreditation of Healthcare Organizations or JCAHO

Joint venture: The result of two or more companies investing together in a mutually beneficial project

Journal entry: An accounting representation of a financial transaction or transfer of amounts between accounts that contains at least one debit and one credit and in which the dollar value of the debits and the credits is the same

Judge-made law: Unwritten law originating from court decisions where no applicable statute exists; *See* **case law; common law**

Judgment sampling: A sampling technique where the researcher relies on his or her own judgment to select the subjects based on relevant expertise

Judicial decision: A ruling handed down by a court to settle a legal matter

Judicial law: The body of law created as a result of court (judicial) decisions

Jurisdiction: The power and authority of a court to hear, interpret, and apply the law to and decide specific types of cases

Justice: The impartial administration of policies or laws that takes into consideration the competing interests and limited resources of the individuals or groups involved

Just-in-time training (JIT): Training provided anytime, anyplace, and just when it is needed

Key: In cryptography, a secret value used to encrypt and decrypt messages; in a symmetric cryptographic algorithm, only one key is needed to encrypt and decrypt a message, but in an asymmetric algorithm, two keys are needed; *See* **cryptography**; **private key**; **public key**

Key attributes: Common fields (attributes) within a relational database that are used to link tables to one another

Key field: An explanatory notation that uniquely identifies each row in a database table; *See* **primary key**

Key indicator: A quantifiable measure used over time to determine whether some structure, process, or outcome in the provision of care to a patient supports high-quality performance measured against best practice criteria

Key performance indicator: Area identified for needed improvement through benchmarking and continuous quality improvement

KMS: *See* **knowledge management system**

K-nearest neighbor (K-NN): A classic technique used to discover associations and sequences when the data attributes are numeric; nonparametric estimator of a function

K-NN: *See* **K-nearest neighbor**

Knowledge: The information, understanding, and experience that give individuals the power to make informed decisions

Knowledge assets: Assets that are the sources of knowledge for an organization (for example, printed documents, unwritten rules, workflows, customer knowledge, data in databases and spreadsheets, and the human expertise, know-how, and tacit knowledge within the minds of the organization's workforce); *Also called* **knowledge-based assets** or **knowledge-based data**

Knowledge base: A database that not only manages raw data but also integrates them with information from various reference works; *See* **data repository**

Knowledge-based assets: *See* **knowledge assets**

Knowledge-based data: *See* **knowledge assets**

Knowledge-based DSS: Decision support system in which the key element is the knowledge base; often referred to as a rule-based system because the knowledge is stored in the form of rules (for example, the IF, THEN, ELSE format)

Knowledge management: 1. The process by which data are acquired and transformed into information through the application of context, which in turn provides understanding 2. A management philosophy that promotes an integrated and collaborative approach to the process of information asset creation, capture, organization, access, and use

Knowledge management system (KMS): A type of system that supports the creation, organization, and dissemination of business or clinical knowledge and expertise to providers, employees, and managers throughout a healthcare enterprise

Knowledge production: Involves the creation of knowledge through collection, generation, synthesis, identification, and organization of knowledge through codification, storage, packaging, and coordination

Knowledge refinement: Consists of evaluation, reflection, adaptation, and sustainability of knowledge

Knowledge sources: Various types of reference material and expert information that are compiled in a manner accessible for integration with patient care information to improve the quality and cost-effectiveness of healthcare provision

Knowledge use: Consists of distribution, sharing, application, and integration of knowledge

Knowledge worker: An employee who improves his or her performance by sharing his or her experience and expertise with other employees

Kolb's "Learning Loop": A theory of experiential learning involving four interrelated steps: concrete experiences, observation and reflection, formation of abstract concepts and theories, and testing new implications of a theory in new situations

Lab panel: A group of tests commonly performed together for a given purpose, usually for one diagnosis

Labeler: Any firm that manufactures, repacks, or distributes a drug product

Labeler Code: The first segment of the National Drug Code (NDC); assigned by FDA to a firm

Labor and delivery record: Health record documentation that takes the place of an operative report for patients who give birth in the obstetrics department of an acute care hospital

Laboratory information system (LIS): An information system that collects, stores, and manages laboratory tests and their respective results. The LIS can speed up access to test results through improved efficiency from various locations, including anywhere in the hospital, the physician's office, or even the clinician's home

Labor-Management Relations Act (Taft-Hartley Act): Federal legislation passed in 1947 that imposed certain restrictions on unions while upholding their right to organize and bargain collectively

Labor-Management Reporting and Disclosure Act (Landrum-Griffin Act): Federal legislation passed in 1959 to ensure that union members' interests were properly represented by union leadership; created, among other things, a bill of rights for union members

Labor organization: *See* **union**

Labor-related share (portion, ratio): Sum of facilities' relative proportion of wages and salaries, employee benefits, professional fees, postal services, other labor-intensive services, and the labor-related share of capital costs from the appropriate market basket. Labor-related share is typically 70 to 75 percent of healthcare facilities' costs. Adjusted annually and published in the *Federal Register*

Labor relations: Human resources management activities associated with unions and collective bargaining

Laggards: A category of adopters of change who are very reluctant to accept proposed changes and may resist transition

LAN: *See* **local-area network**

Language translator: A software system that translates a program written in a particular computer language into a language that other types of computers can understand

Large urban area: An urban area with a population of more than one million

Laser: A tool such as the argon laser and the Nd:YAG laser used to cut or destroy tissue; acronym for light amplification by stimulated emission of radiation

Late enrollee: Individual who does not enroll in a group healthcare plan at the first opportunity, but enrolls later if the plan has a general open enrollment period

Late entry: An addition to the health record when a pertinent entry was missed or was not written in a timely manner

Late fetal death: The death of a product of human conception that is 28 weeks or more of gestation and weighs 1,001 grams or more before its complete expulsion or extraction from the mother

Late majority: Skeptical group that comprises another 34 percent of the organization: individuals in this group usually adopt innovations only after social or financial pressure to do so

LBW: Low birth weight

LCD: *See* **local coverage determination**

LCMS: *See* **Learning Content Management System**

Leader–member exchange: Micro theory that focuses on dyadic relationships, or those between two people or between a leader and a small group; explains how in-group and out-group relationships form with a leader or mentor, and how delegation may occur

Leader–member relations: Group atmosphere much like social orientation; includes the subordinates' acceptance of, and confidence in, the leader as well as the loyalty and commitment they show toward the leader

Leadership grid: Blake and Mouton's grid that marked off degrees of emphasis toward orientation using a nine-point scale and finally separated the grid into five styles of management based on the combined people and production emphasis

Leading: One of the four management functions in which people are directed and motivated to achieve goals

Leapfrog Group: Organization that promotes healthcare safety by giving consumers the information they need to make better-informed choices about the hospitals they choose

Learning Content Management System (LCMS): Training software development tools that assist with management, sharing, and reuse of course content

Learning curve: The time required to acquire and apply certain skills so that new levels of productivity and/or performance exceed prelearning levels (productivity often is inversely related to the learning curve)

Learning Management System (LMS): A software application that assists with managing and tracking learners and learning events and collating data on learner progress

Learning organization: An organization in which the emphasis is on acquiring and sharing business knowledge along with delivering information quickly, clearly, and visually to everyone within the organization

Least-Preferred Coworker Scale (LPC): Presents a series of 16 to 22 bipolar adjectives along an eight-point rating scale; sample items include unfriendly to friendly, uncooperative to cooperative, and hostile to supportive

Leave of absence: The authorized absence of an inpatient from a hospital or other facility for a specified period of time occurring after admission and prior to discharge

Leave of absence day: A day occurring after the admission and prior to the discharge of a hospital inpatient when the patient is not present at the census-taking hour because he or she is on a leave of absence from the healthcare facility

Lecture: A one-way method of delivering education through speaking in which the teacher delivers the speech and the student listens

LEEP: loop electrode excision procedure

Legacy system: A type of computer system that uses older technology but may still perform optimally

Legal electronic health record: Data or other digital information that exists in an electronic system and provides evidence of what happened. A subset of documents or data in the EHR used for evidence

Legal entity: The form of a business organization recognized by law, for example, a sole proprietorship, a partnership, or a corporation

Legal health record (LHR): Documents and data elements that a healthcare provider may include in response to legally permissible requests for patient information

Legal hold: A communication issued because of current or anticipated litigation, audit, government investigation, or other such matters that suspend the normal disposition or processing of records. Legal holds can encompass business procedures affecting active data, including, but not limited to, backup tape recycling. The specific communication to business or IT organizations may also be called a "hold," "preservation order," "suspension order," "freeze notice," "hold order," or "hold notice."

Legibility: An aspect of the quality of provider entries in which an entry or notation is readable

Legislative law: *See* **statutory law**

Length of stay (LOS): The total number of patient days for an inpatient episode, calculated by subtracting the date of admission from the date of discharge

Level of service: 1. The relative intensity of services given when a physician provides one-on-one services for a patient (such as minimal, brief, limited, or intermediate) 2. The relative intensity of services provided by a healthcare facility (for example, tertiary care); *Also called* **level of significance**

Level of significance: *See* **level of service**

Leveraged buyout: The result of the stock of a publicly traded company being purchased, often by its own management, with a large amount of debt and the company's assets as collateral for the loan

Lexicon: 1. The vocabulary used in a language or a subject area or by a particular speaker or group of speakers 2. A collection of words or terms and their meanings for a particular domain, used in healthcare for drug terms

LHR: *See* **legal health record**

Liability: 1. A legal obligation or responsibility that may have financial repercussions if not fulfilled 2. An amount owed by an individual or organization to another individual or organization

Liability files policy: A policy that outlines procedures for limiting access to, and maintaining the security of, information related to liability cases

License: The legal authorization granted by a state to an entity that allows the entity to provide healthcare services within a specific scope of services and geographical location; states license both individual healthcare professionals and healthcare facilities; licensure usually requires an applicant to pass an examination to obtain the license initially and then to participate in continuing education activities to maintain the license thereafter

Licensed independent practitioner: Any individual permitted by law to provide healthcare services without direction or supervision, within the scope of the individual's license as conferred by state regulatory agencies and consistent with individually granted clinical privileges

Licensed practitioner: An individual at any level of professional specialization who requires a public license or certification to engage in patient care

Licensure: The legal authority or formal permission from authorities to carry on certain activities that by law or regulation require such permission (applicable to institutions as well as individuals)

Licensure requirements: Criteria healthcare providers must meet in order to gain and retain state licensure to provide specific services

Life cycle costs: The costs of a project beyond its purchase price, for example, setup costs, maintenance costs, training costs, and so on, as well as costs incurred throughout the project's estimated useful life

Likert scale: An ordinal scaling and summated rating technique for measuring the attitudes of respondents; a measure that records level of agreement or disagreement along a progression of categories, usually five (five-point scale), often administered in the form of a questionnaire

Limitation: Qualification or other specification that reduces or restricts the extent of a healthcare benefit

Limited data set: PHI that excludes direct identifiers of the individual and the individual's relatives, employers, or household members but still does not deidentify the information

Limiting charge: A percentage limit on physicians' fees that nonparticipating providers may bill Medicare beneficiaries above the fee schedule amount

Linear programming: An operational management technique that uses mathematical formulas to determine the optimal way to allocate resources for a project

Line authority: The authority to manage subordinates and to have them report back, based on relationships illustrated in an organizational chart

Line chart: A type of data display tool used to plot information on the progress of a process over time

Line graph: A graphic technique used to illustrate the relationship between continuous measurements; consists of a line drawn to connect a series of points on an arithmetic scale; often used to display time trends

Line item: A service- or item-specific detail of a budget, bill, or reimbursement claim

Linkage analysis: A technique used to explore and examine relationships among a large number of variables of different types

Linking: The assignment of diagnosis codes to individual line items (1 through 4) on a CMS-1500 claim form to cross-reference the procedure to the diagnosis code, establishing the medical necessity of the procedure

Linux: A freeware operating system similar to UNIX

Liquidity: The degree to which assets can be quickly and efficiently turned into cash, for example, marketable securities are generally liquid, the assumption being that they can be sold for their full value in a matter of days, whereas buildings are not liquid, because they cannot usually be sold quickly

LIS: *See* **laboratory information system**

Literature review: A systematic investigation of all the knowledge available about a topic from sources such as books, journal articles, theses, and dissertations; *See* **systematic literature review**

Litigation: A civil lawsuit or contest in court

Living arrangement: A data element that denotes whether the patient lives alone or with others

Living will: A directive that allows an individual to describe in writing the type of healthcare that he or she would or would not wish to receive

LMRPs: *See* **local medical review policies**

LMS: *See* **Learning Management System**

Local-area network (LAN): A network that connects multiple computer devices via continuous cable within a relatively small geographic area

Local Coverage Determination (LCD): New format for LMRPs: Coverage rules, at a fiscal intermediary (FI) or carrier level, that provide information on what diagnoses justify the medical necessity of a test; LCDs vary from state to state

Local medical review policies (LMRPs): Documents that define Medicare coverage of outpatient services via lists of diagnoses defined as medically reasonable and necessary for the services provided; *See* **Local Coverage Determination (LCD)**

Location or address of encounter: The full address and nine-digit zip code for the location at which outpatient care was received from the healthcare practitioner of record

Locked: The process by which a health record entry is complete and any changes to the entry must be made through an amendment

Logical: 1. A user's view of the way data or systems are organized (for example, a file that is a collection of data stored together) 2. The opposite of physical

Logical data model: The second level of data model that is drawn according to the type of database to be developed

Logical Observation Identifiers, Names and Codes (LOINC): A database protocol developed by the Regenstrief Institute for Health Care aimed at standardizing laboratory and clinical codes for use in clinical care, outcomes management, and research

Logical (or conceptual) repository: The compilation of multiple physical repositories

LOINC: *See* **Logical Observation Identifiers, Names and Codes**

Longitudinal: A type of time frame for research studies during which data are collected from the same participants at multiple points in time

Longitudinal health record: A permanent, coordinated patient record of significant information listed in chronological order and maintained across time, ideally from birth to death

Long-term assets: Assets whose value to the organization extends beyond one fiscal year, for example, buildings, land, and equipment are long-term assets; *See* **fixed assets**

Long-term care: Healthcare services provided in a non-acute care setting to chronically ill, aged, disabled, or mentally handicapped individuals

Long-term care diagnosis related group (LTC-DRG): Inpatient classification that categorizes patients who are similar in terms of diagnoses and treatments, age, resources used, and lengths of stay. Under the prospective payment system (PPS), hospitals are paid a set fee for treating patients in a single DRG category, regardless of the actual cost of care for the individual. LTC-DRGs are exactly the same as the DRGs for the inpatient prospective payment system (IPPS). *See also* **diagnosis related group (DRG)**

Long-term care facility: A healthcare organization that provides medical, nursing, rehabilitation, and subacute care services to residents who need continual supervision and/or assistance

Long-term care hospital (LTCH): According to the Centers for Medicare and Medicaid Services (CMS), a hospital with an average length of stay for Medicare patients that is 25 days or longer, or a hospital excluded from the inpatient prospective payment system and that has an average length of stay for all patients that is 20 days or longer

LOS: *See* **length of stay**

Loss prevention: A risk management strategy that includes developing and revising policies and procedures that are both facility-wide and department specific

Loss reduction: A component of a risk management program that encompasses techniques used to manage events or claims that already have taken place

Low-birth-weight neonate: Any newborn baby, regardless of gestational age, whose birth weight is less than 2,500 grams

Low-utilization payment adjustment (LUPA): An alternative (reduced) payment made to home health agencies instead of the home health resource group reimbursement rate when a patient receives fewer than four home care visits during a 60-day episode

Low-volume hospital: A hospital with fewer than 200 discharges per fiscal year and located more than 25 miles from the nearest hospital

Lower courts: The lowest level of the US judicial system, where state and local criminal and civil cases are tried; *See* **trial courts**

LPC: *See* **Least-Preferred Coworker Scale**

LTCH: *See* **inpatient long-term care hospital**

Lumper Vocabulary: A medical vocabulary that does not attempt to provide names for all things and activities, but rather provides codes that combine multiple concepts for a specific purpose; for example, LOINC gathers concepts into a code that can be "exploded" into components when needed

LUPA: *See* **low-utilization payment adjustment**

MAC: Monitored anesthesia care; *See also* **maximum allowable charges**; **Medicare administrative contractor**

Machine language: Binary codes made up of zeroes and ones that computers use directly to represent precise storage locations and operations

Machine learning: An area of computer science that studies algorithms and computer programs that improve employee performance on some task by exposure to a training or learning experience

Macro virus: A type of computer virus that infects Microsoft Word or similar applications by inserting unwanted words or phrases; most are relatively harmless

Magnetic resonance image (MRI): The generation of a powerful magnetic field that surrounds the patient, creating computer-interpreted radio frequency imaging

Mainframe: A computer architecture built with a single central processing unit to which dumb terminals and/or personal computers are connected

Mainframe architecture: The term used to refer to the configuration of a mainframe computer; *See* **mainframe**

Main provider: A provider that either creates or owns another entity in order to deliver additional healthcare services under its name, ownership, and financial and administrative control

Maintenance and evaluation phase: The fourth and final phase of the systems development life cycle that helps to ensure that adequate technical support staff and resources are available to maintain or support the new system

Major diagnostic category (MDC): Under diagnosis-related groups (DRGs), one of 25 categories based on single or multiple organ systems into which all diseases and disorders relating to that system are classified

Major drug class: A general therapeutic or pharmacological classification scheme for prescription drug products reported to the Food and Drug Administration under the provisions of the Drug Listing Act

Major medical insurance: Prepaid healthcare benefits that include a high limit for most types of medical expenses and usually require a large deductible and sometimes place limits on coverage and charges (for example, room and board); *Also called* **catastrophic coverage**

Major teaching hospital: A hospital that provides clinical education to 100 or more resident physicians

Malfeasance: A wrong or improper act

Malpractice (MP), medical malpractice: 1. The improper or negligent treatment of a patient, as by a physician, resulting in injury, damage, or loss 2. Element of the relative value unit (RVU): costs of the premiums for professional liability insurance 3. The professional liability of healthcare providers in the delivery of patient care

Managed behavioral healthcare organization (MBHO): A type of healthcare organization that delivers and manages all aspects of behavioral healthcare or the payment for care by limiting providers of care, discounting payment to providers of care, and/or limiting access to care

Managed care: 1. Payment method in which the third-party payer has implemented some provisions to control the costs of healthcare while maintaining quality care 2. Systematic merger of clinical, financial, and administrative processes to mange access, cost, and quality of healthcare

Managed care organization (MCO): A type of healthcare organization that delivers medical care and manages all aspects of the care or the payment for care by limiting providers of care, discounting payment to providers of care, and/or limiting access to care; *Also called* coordinated care organization

Managed fee-for-service reimbursement: A healthcare plan that implements utilization controls (prospective and retrospective review of healthcare services) for reimbursement under traditional fee-for-service insurance plans

Management: The process of planning, organizing, and leading organizational activities

Management by objectives (MBO): A management approach that defines target objectives for organizing work and compares performance against those objectives

Management functions: Traditionally, the tasks of planning, organizing, directing, coordinating, and controlling

Management information system (MIS): A computer-based system that provides information to a healthcare organization's managers for use in making decisions that affect a variety of day-to-day activities

Management of Information (IM): One chapter of the Joint Commission's *Comprehensive Accreditation Manual for Hospitals (CAMH)* that promulgates the Joint Commission's requirements regarding the data and information used for various purposes in hospital organizations

Management services organization (MSO): An organization, usually owned by a group of physicians or a hospital, that provides administrative and support services to one or more physician group practices or small hospitals

Management support information systems: Systems that provide information primarily to support manager decision making

Managerial accounting: The development, implementation, and analysis of systems that track financial transactions for management control purposes, including both budget systems and cost analysis systems

Many-to-many relationship: The concept (occurring only in a conceptual model) that multiple instances of an entity may be associated with multiple instances of another entity

Map: 1. Locating the route of passage of electrical impulses and/or locating functional areas in a body part. It is only applicable to the cardiac conduction mechanism and the central nervous system 2. The process of identifying equivalent terms or concepts in two different classifications or vocabulary systems

Mapping: Creation of a cross map that links the content from one classification or terminology scheme to another

Marital status: The marital state of the patient at the start of care (for example, married, living together, not living together, never married, widowed, divorced, separated, or unknown/not stated)

Market basket: Mix of goods and services for a particular market

Market basket index: Relative measure that averages the costs of a mix of goods and services; used in the home health prospective payment system to reflect changes over time in the prices of an appropriate mix of goods and services and to develop the national 60-day episode payment rates

Marketing: The process of issuing a communication about a product or service with the purpose of encouraging recipients of the communication to purchase or use the product or service

Market value: The price at which something can be bought or sold on the open market

Mark sense technology: Technology that detects the presence or absence of hand-marked characters on analog documents; used for processing questionnaires, surveys, and tests, such as filled-in circles by Number 2 pencils on exam forms

MARs: *See* **medication administration records**

Maslow's Hierarchy of Needs: A theory developed by Abraham Maslow suggesting that a hierarchy of needs might help explain behavior and guide managers on how to motivate employees; *See* **hierarchy of needs**

Massachusetts General Hospital Utility Multiprogramming System: *See* **M technology**

Massed training: An educational technique that requires learning a large amount of material at one time

Master patient index (MPI): A patient-identifying directory referencing all patients related to an organization and which also serves as a link to the patient record or information, facilitates patient identification, and assists in maintaining a longitudinal patient record from birth to death; *See* **master person index**; **master population index**

Master person index: *See* **master patient index**

Master population index: *See* **master patient index**

Master resident index: A listing or database that a long-term care facility keeps to record all the residents who have ever been admitted or treated there

Master resident index maintenance policy: A policy that outlines procedures on the maintenance of the master resident index and the steps to take to verify and cross-check all entries

Matching: A concept that enables decision makers to look at expenses and revenues in the same period to measure the organization's income performance

Matching expenses: The costs that are recorded during the same period as the related revenue

Materiality: The significance of a dollar amount based on predetermined criteria

Materials management system: Information system that manages the supplies and equipment within a facility

Material safety data sheet (MSDS): Documentation maintained on the hazardous materials used in a healthcare organization. The documentation outlines such information as common and chemical names, family name, and product codes; risks associated with the material, including overall health risk, flammability, reactivity with other chemicals, and effects at the site of contact; descriptions of the protective equipment and clothing that should be used to handle the material; and other similar information

Maternal death: The death of any woman, from any cause, related to or aggravated by pregnancy or its management (regardless of duration or site of pregnancy), but not from accidental or incidental causes

Maternal death rate (hospital based): For a hospital, the total number of maternal deaths directly related to pregnancy for a given time period divided by the total number of obstetrical discharges for the same time period; for a community, the total number of deaths attributed to maternal conditions during a given time period in a specific geographic area divided by the total number of live births for the same time period in the same area

Maternal mortality rate (community based): A rate that measures the deaths associated with pregnancy for a specific community for a specific period of time

Maximum allowable charges (MAC): The maximum charges allowed for a service rendered

Maximum out-of-pocket cost: Specific amount, in a certain time frame such as one year, beyond which all covered healthcare services for that policyholder or dependent are paid at 100 percent by the healthcare insurance plan; *See* **catastrophic expense limit; stop-loss benefit**

MBHO: *See* **managed behavioral healthcare organization**

MBO: *See* **management by objectives**

MCO: *See* **managed care organization**

MDC: *See* **major diagnostic category**

MDDBMS: *See* **multidimensional database management system**

MDM: *See* **medical decision making**

MDS: *See* **Minimum Data Set**

MDS-PAC: *See* **Minimum Data Set for Post Acute Care**

MDS processing policy: A policy that applies when health record personnel are included in the MDS data entry or submission of the MDS data

MDS 2.0: *See* **Minimum Data Set for Long-Term Care, Version 2.0**

Mean: A measure of central tendency that is determined by calculating the arithmetic average of the observations in a frequency distribution

Meaningful Use: A regulation that was issued by the Centers for Medicare and Medicaid Services (CMS) on July 28, 2010, outlining an incentive program for professionals (EPs), eligible hospitals, and critical access hospitals (CAHs) participating in Medicare and Medicaid programs that adopt and successfully demonstrate meaningful use of certified electronic health record (EHR) technology

Meaningful use of certified EHRs: Under ARRA, the term meaningful use refers to use of an EHR according to published criteria. Certified EHR means certification by an accreditation body, of which CCHIT was the first. The phrase "meaningful use of certified EHR" is used in reference to the criteria set out in ARRA by which a hospital or eligible professional can receive incentive funding from Medicare or Medicaid for appropriate use of a well-functioned electronic health record system

Measure: The quantifiable data about a function or process

Measurement: The systematic process of data collection, repeated over time or at a single point in time

Measures of central tendency: The typical or average numbers that are descriptive of the entire collection of data for a specific population

MEDCIN®: A proprietary clinical terminology developed as a point-of-care tool for electronic medical record documentation at the time and place of patient care

MedDRA: *See* **Medical Dictionary for Regulatory Activities**

Media controls: The policies and procedures that govern the receipt, storage, and removal of hardware, software, and computer media (such as disks and tapes) into and out of the organization

Median: A measure of central tendency that shows the midpoint of a frequency distribution when the observations have been arranged in order from lowest to highest

Mediation: In law, when a dispute is submitted to a third party to facilitate agreement between the disputing parties

Medicaid: An entitlement program that oversees medical assistance for individuals and families with low incomes and limited resources; jointly funded between state and federal governments and legislated by the Social Security Act

Medicaid Integrity Contract (MIC): CMS contracts with eligible entities to review and audit Medicaid claims to identify overpayments and provide education on program integrity issues

Medical audits: *See* **medical care evaluation studies**

Medical care evaluation studies: Audits required by the Medicare Conditions of Participation that dictate the use of screening criteria with evaluation by diagnosis and/or procedure; *Also called* **medical audits**

Medical care unit: An assemblage of inpatient beds (or newborn bassinets), related facilities, and assigned personnel that provide service to a defined and limited class of patients according to their particular medical care needs

Medical classification system: A method of arranging related diseases and conditions into groups to be reported as quantitative data for statistical purposes

Medical consultation: *See* **consultation**

Medical Data Interchange Standard (MEDIX): A set of hospital system interface transaction standards developed by the Institute of Electrical and Electronics Engineers

Medical decision making: The process of establishing a diagnosis and/or management option for a patient

Medical device reporting: The Food and Drug Administration (FDA) requires reporting of deaths and severe complications thought to be due to a device to the FDA and the manufacturer

Medical Dictionary for Regulatory Activities (MedDRA): A vocabulary that has been developed within the regulatory environment as a pragmatic, clinically validated medical terminology with an emphasis on ease-of-use data entry, retrieval, analysis, and display, with a suitable balance between sensitivity and specificity

Medical emergency: Severe injury or illness (including pain) in need of immediate medical attention; definition depends upon healthcare insurer

Medical examiner: Typically a physician with pathology training given the responsibility by a government, such as a county or state, for investigating suspicious deaths

Medical foundation: Multipurpose, nonprofit service organization for physicians and other healthcare providers at the local and county level; as managed care organizations, medical foundations have established preferred provider organizations, exclusive provider organizations, and management service organizations, with emphases on freedom of choice and preservation of the physician–patient relationship

Medical Group Management Association (MGMA): A national organization composed of individuals actively engaged in the business management of medical groups consisting of three or more physicians in medical practice

Medical history: A record of previous information provided by a patient to his or her physician to explain the patient's chief complaint, present and past illnesses, and personal and family medical problems; includes also medications and health risk factors

Medical home: A program to provide comprehensive primary care that partners physicians with the patient and their family to allow better access to healthcare and improved outcomes; *Also called* **Patient-Centered Medical Home (PCMH)**

Medical informatics: A field of information science concerned with the management of data and information used to diagnose, treat, cure, and prevent disease through the application of computers and computer technologies

Medical informatics professionals: Individuals who work in the field of medical informatics

Medical information bus (MIB): The part of the IEEE standard that provides open integration standards for connecting electronic patient-monitoring devices with information systems

**Medical Literature Analysis and Retrieval System Online
(MEDLINE):** A computerized, online database in
the bibliographic Medical Literature Analysis and
Retrieval System (MEDLARS) of the National Library
of Medicine

Medical malpractice: A type of action in which the plaintiff
must demonstrate that a healthcare provider-patient
relationship existed at the time of the alleged wrongful act

Medical malpractice insurance: Insurance that protects a
party from claims for medical negligence or other tor-
tuous injury arising out of care provided to patients

Medical necessity: 1. The likelihood that a proposed healthcare service will have a reasonable beneficial effect on
the patient's physical condition and quality of life at a
specific point in his or her illness or lifetime 2. Healthcare services and supplies that are proven or acknowl-
edged to be effective in the diagnosis, treatment, cure,
or relief of a health condition, illness, injury, disease,
or its symptoms and to be consistent with the community's accepted standard of care. Under medical
necessity, only those services, procedures, and patient
care warranted by the patient's condition are provided
3. The concept that procedures are only eligible for
reimbursement as a covered benefit when they are performed for a specific diagnosis or specified frequency;
Also called **need-to-know principle**

Medical nomenclature: A recognized system of preferred
terminology for naming disease processes

Medical Outcomes Study Short-Form Health Survey: A
patient survey that reflects the patients' disease and
symptom intensity to characterize the total burden of
the disease

Medical record: *See* **health record**

Medical record administrator: *See* **health information
management professional**

Medical records department: *See* **health information services department**

Medical record entry: *See* **health record entry**

Medical record number: *See* **health record number**

Medical record technician: *See* **health information management professional**

Medical research: *See* **clinical research**

Medical savings account (MSA) plans: Plans that provide benefits after a single, high deductible has been met whereby Medicare makes an annual deposit to the MSA and the beneficiary is expected to use the money in the MSA to pay for medical expenses below the annual deductible

Medical services: The activities relating to medical care performed by physicians, nurses, and other healthcare professional and technical personnel under the direction of a physician

Medical specialties: A group of clinical specialties that concentrates on the provision of nonsurgical care by physicians who have received advanced training in internal medicine, pediatrics, cardiology, endocrinology, psychiatry, oncology, nephrology, neurology, pulmonology, gastroenterology, dermatology, radiology, and nuclear medicine, among many other concentrations

Medical staff: The staff members of a healthcare organization who are governed by medical staff bylaws; may or may not be employed by the healthcare organization

Medical staff bylaws: Standards governing the practice of medical staff members; typically voted upon by the organized medical staff and the medical staff executive committee and approved by the facility's board; governs the business conduct, rights, and responsibilities of the medical staff; medical staff members must abide by these bylaws in order to continue practice in the healthcare facility

Medical staff classifications: Categories of clinical practice privileges assigned to individual practitioners on the basis of their qualifications; *See* **medical staff privileges**

Medical staff executive committee: A body composed of those elected representative members of the medical staff who are authorized to act on behalf of the medical staff

Medical staff organization (MSO): A self-governing entity that operates as a responsible extension of the governing body and exists for the purpose of providing patient care

Medical staff privileges: Categories of clinical practice privileges assigned to individual practitioners on the basis of their qualifications

Medical staff unit: One of the departments, divisions, or specialties into which the organized medical staff of a hospital is divided

Medical Subjects Heading database (MeSH): The National Library of Medicine's (NLM's) controlled vocabulary for indexing journal articles

Medical transcription: The conversion of verbal medical reports dictated by healthcare providers into written form for inclusion in patients' health records

Medical transcriptionist: A medical language specialist who types or word-processes information dictated by providers into written form

Medical vocabulary: *See* **clinical vocabulary**

Medically needy option: An option in the Medicaid program that allows states to extend eligibility to persons who would be eligible for Medicaid under one of the mandatory or optional groups but whose income and/ or resources fall above the eligibility level set by their state

Medically Unlikely Edits (MUEs): A unit of service for HCPCS/CPT codes submitted by a single provider or supplier to a single beneficiary on the same date of service; implemented in 2007 to reduce the paid claim error rate for Part B claims

Medicare: A federally funded health program established in 1965 to assist with the medical care costs of Americans 65 years of age and older as well as other individuals entitled to Social Security benefits owing to their disabilities

Medicare administrative contractor (MAC): Newly established contracting entities that will administer Medicare Part A and Part B as of 2011; MACs will replace the carriers and fiscal intermediaries

Medicare Advantage (Medicare Part C): Optional managed care plan for Medicare beneficiaries who are entitled to Part A, enrolled in Part B, and live in an area with a plan; types include health maintenance organization, point-of-service plan, preferred provider organization, and provider-sponsored organization

Medicare carrier: A health plan that processes Part B claims for services by physicians and medical suppliers (for example, the Blue Shield plan in a state)

Medicare Conditions of Participation (COP) or Conditions for Coverage: A publication that describes the requirements that institutional providers (such as hospitals, skilled nursing facilities, and home health agencies) must meet to receive reimbursement for services provided to Medicare beneficiaries

Medicare discharge: The status of Medicare patients who are formally released from a hospital, die in a hospital, or are transferred to another hospital or unit excluded from the prospective payment system

Medicare economic index (MEI): An index used by the Medicare program to update physician fee levels in relation to annual changes in the general economy for inflation, productivity, and changes in specific health-sector expense factors including malpractice, personnel costs, rent, and other expenses

Medicare fee schedule (MFS): A feature of the resource-based relative value system that includes a complete list of the payments Medicare makes to physicians and other providers

Medicare Modernization Act of 2003 (MMA): Legislation passed in 2003 designed to expand healthcare services for seniors, with a major focus on prescription drug benefits

Medicare nonparticipation: The status with the Medicare program in which the provider has not signed a participation agreement and does not accept the Medicare allowable fee as payment in full, with the result that the payment goes directly to the patient and the patient must pay the bill up to Medicare's limiting charge of 115% of the approved amount

Medicare Part A: The portion of Medicare that provides benefits for inpatient hospital services; *See* **hospitalization insurance**

Medicare Part B: An optional and supplemental portion of Medicare that provides benefits for physician services, medical services, and medical supplies not covered by Medicare Part A; *See* **supplemental medical insurance**

Medicare Part C: A managed care option that includes services under Parts A, B, and D and additional services that are not typically covered by Medicare; Medicare Part C requires an additional premium; *See* **Medicare Advantage**

Medicare Part D: Medicare drug benefit created by the Medicare Modernization Act of 2003 (MMA) that offers outpatient drug coverage to beneficiaries for an additional premium

Medicare participation: The status with the Medicare program in which the provider signs a participation agreement with Medicare and agrees to accept the allowable fee as payment in full and the patient pays any remaining balance, up to the allowed fee

Medicare prospective payment system: The reimbursement system for inpatient hospital services provided to Medicare and Medicaid beneficiaries that is based on the use of diagnosis-related groups (DRGs) as a classification tool; *See* **acute care prospective payment system; home health prospective payment system; skilled nursing facility prospective payment system**

Medicare Provider Analysis and Review (MEDPAR) database system: A database containing information and files submitted by fiscal intermediaries that is used by the Office of the Inspector General to identify suspicious billing and charge practices

Medicare Provider Analysis and Review (MEDPAR) File: A database containing information submitted by fiscal intermediaries that is used by the Office of the Inspector General to identity suspicious billing and charge practices

Medicare-required assessment: A Minimum Data Set for Long-Term Care completed solely for the purpose of Medicare rate setting for skilled nursing facilities

Medicare secondary payer: One of the edits in the outpatient and inpatient code editors that reviews claims to determine if the claim should be paid by another form of insurance, such as workers' compensation or private insurance in the event of a traffic accident

Medicare severity diagnosis-related groups (MS-DRGs): The US government's 2007 revision of the DRG system, the MS-DRG system better accounts for severity of illness and resource consumption

Medicare summary notice (MSN): A summary sent to the patient from Medicare that summarizes all services provided over a period of time with an explanation of benefits provided

Medicare volume performance standard (MVPS): A goal to control the annual rate of growth in Part B expenditures for physicians' services

Medication administration records (MARs): The records used to document the date and time each dose and type of medication is administered to a patient

Medication administration system: Information system designed to support the administration of medications safely

Medication error: A mistake that involves an accidental drug overdose, an administration of an incorrect substance, an accidental consumption of a drug, or a misuse of a drug or biological during a medical or surgical procedure

Medication list: An ongoing record of the medications a patient has received in the past and is taking currently; includes names of medications, dosages, amounts dispensed, dispensing instructions, prescription dates, discontinued dates, and the problem for which the medication was prescribed

Medications prescribed: Descriptions (including, where possible, the National Drug Code, dosage, strength, and total amount prescribed) of all medications prescribed or provided by the healthcare practitioner at the encounter (for outpatients) or given on discharge to the patient (for inpatients)

Medication reconciliation: Process that monitors and confirms that the patient receives consistent dosing across all facility transfers, such as on admission, from nursing unit to surgery, and from surgery to intensive care unit (ICU)

Medication record: Health record documentation that lists all of the medications administered to a patient while he or she is on a nursing unit

Medication usage review: An evaluation of medication use and medication processes

Medigap: A private insurance policy that supplements Medicare coverage

MEDIX: *See* **Medical Data Interchange Standard**

MEDLINE: *See* **Medical Literature Analysis and Retrieval System Online**

MEDPAR database system: *See* **Medicare Provider Analysis and Review database system**

MEDPAR File: *See* **Medicare Provider Analysis and Review File**

MEI: *See* **Medicare economic index**

Member: Individual or entity that purchases healthcare insurance coverage *See* **certificate holder; insured; policyholder; subscriber**

Member months: The total membership each month accumulated for a given time period (for example, 100 members serviced each month for six months equals 600 member months)

Mental ability (cognitive) tests: Examinations that assess the reasoning capabilities of individuals

Mentor: A trusted advisor or counselor; an experienced individual who educates and trains another individual within an occupational setting

Mentoring: A type of coaching and training in which an individual is matched with a more experienced individual who serves as an advisor or counselor

Merger: A business situation where two or more companies combine, but one of them continues to exist as a legal business entity while the others cease to exist legally and their assets and liabilities become part of the continuing company

MeSH: *See* **Medical Subjects Heading database**

Message format standards: Protocols that help ensure that data transmitted from one system to another remain comparable; *See* **data exchange standards**

Messaging standards: *See* **transmission standards**

Meta-analysis: A specialized form of systematic literature review that involves the statistical analysis of a large collection of results from individual studies for the purpose of integrating the studies' findings

Metadata: Descriptive data that characterize other data to create a clearer understanding of their meaning and to achieve greater reliability and quality of information. Metadata consist of both indexing terms and attributes. Data about data: for example, creation date, date sent, date received, last access date, last modification date

MetamorphoSys: The installation wizard and customization program included in each release of the Unified Medical Language System

Metathesaurus®: The very large, multipurpose, and multilingual vocabulary database that is the central vocabulary component of the Unified Medical Language System

Method: 1. A way of performing an action or task 2. A strategy used by a researcher to collect, analyze, and present data

Metropolitan division: County or group of counties within a core-based statistical area (CBSA) that contains a core with a population of at least 2.5 million. A metropolitan division consists of one or more main or secondary counties that represent an employment center or centers, plus adjacent counties associated with the main county or counties through commuting ties; *See* **core-based statistical area**

Metropolitan statistical area (MSA): Core-based statistical area associated with at least one urbanized area that has a population of at least 50,000. The MSA comprises the central county or counties containing the core, plus adjacent outlying counties; *See* **core-based statistical area**

MFS: *See* **Medicare fee schedule**

MGMA: *See* **Medical Group Management Association**

MIB: *See* **medical information bus**

MIC: *See* **Medicaid Integrity Contract**

Microcomputer: A personal computer characterized by its relatively small size and fast processing speed; *Also called* desktop computer; laptop computer; PC

Microcontroller: A small, low-cost computer (embedded chip) installed in an appliance or electronic device to perform a specific task or program

Microfilming: A photographic process that reduces an original paper document into a small image on film to save storage space

Middle digit filing system: A numeric filing system in which the middle digits are used as the finding aid to organize the filing system

Middle management: The management level in an organization that is concerned primarily with facilitating the work performed by supervisory- and staff-level personnel as well as by executive leaders

Middle managers: The individuals in an organization who oversee the operation of a broad scope of functions at the departmental level or who oversee defined product or service lines

Middleware: A bridge between two applications or the software equivalent of an interface

Midnight rule: A Medicare regulation that states the day preceding a leave of absence becomes a nonbillable day for Medicare purposes when a Part A beneficiary takes a leave of absence and is not present in the skilled nursing facility at midnight

Midsize computer: *See* **minicomputer**

Migration path: A series of coordinated and planned steps required to move a plan from one situation level to another

Milestone budget: A type of budget without a fixed 12-month calendar in which cost is determined and budget allocation is established for the next period as events are completed; *See* **program budget**

MIME: *See* **multipurpose Internet mail extension**

Minicomputer: A small mainframe computer

Minimum Data Set for Long-Term Care Version 2.0 (MDS 2.0): A federally mandated standard assessment form that Medicare- and/or Medicaid-certified nursing facilities must use to collect demographic and clinical data on nursing home residents; includes screening, clinical, and functional status elements

Minimum Data Set for Post Acute Care (MDS-PAC): A patient-centered assessment instrument that must be completed for every Medicare patient, which emphasizes a patient's care needs instead of provider characteristics

Minimum necessary standard: A stipulation of the HIPAA Privacy Rule that requires healthcare facilities and other covered entities to make reasonable efforts to limit the patient-identifiable information they disclose to the least amount required to accomplish the intended purpose for which the information was requested

Minor: An individual who is under the age of majority (usually 18 years of age) who has not been legally emancipated (declared an adult) by the court

Minutes: The written record of key events in a formal meeting

Mirrored processing: The act of entering data into a primary and a secondary server simultaneously so that the secondary server can continue to process the data in the event the primary server crashes

MIS: *See* **management information system**

Miscellaneous codes: National codes used when a supplier is submitting a bill for an item or service where no national code exists to describe the item or service being billed

Misdemeanor: A crime that is less serious than a felony

Misfeasance: Relating to negligence or improper performance during an otherwise correct act

Mission statement: A written statement that sets forth the core purpose and philosophies of an organization or group; defines the organization or group's general purpose for existing

Mitigation: The Privacy Rule (45 CFR 164.530(f)) requires covered entities to lessen, as much as possible, harmful effects that result from the wrongful use and disclosure of protected health information. Possible courses of action may include an apology; disciplinary action against the responsible employee or employees (although such results will not be able to be shared with the wronged individual); repair of the process that resulted in the breach; payment of a bill or financial loss that resulted from the infraction; or gestures of goodwill and good public relations, such as a gift certificate, that may assuage the individual

Mixed costs: Costs that are part variable and part fixed

m-learning: Mobile learning; the application of e-learning to mobile computing devices and wireless networks; *See* **e-learning**

MMA: *See* **Medicare Modernization Act of 2003**

Mode: A measure of central tendency that consists of the most frequent observation in a frequency distribution

Model: The representation of a theory in a visual format, on a smaller scale, or with objects

Model-based DDS: Decision support system that attempts to include as many different models as can be accommodated to provide the user the greatest flexibility in framing the decision situation

Modifier: A two-digit numeric code listed after a procedure code that indicates that a service was altered in some way from the stated CPT descriptor without changing the definition; also used to enhance a code narrative to describe the circumstances of each procedure or service and how it individually applies to a patient

Mohs' micrographic surgery: A type of surgery performed to remove complex or ill-defined skin cancer, requiring a single physician to act in two integrated, but separate and distinct, capacities: surgeon and pathologist

MOLAP: *See* **multidimensional online analytical processing**

Monitoring stage: In performance management, the stage during which established performance standards are continuously checked for any additional need corrections

Morality: A composite of the personal values concerning what is considered right or wrong in a specific cultural group

Moral values: A system of principles by which one guides one's life, usually with regard to right or wrong

Morbidity: The state of being diseased (including illness, injury, or deviation from normal health); the number of sick persons or cases of disease in relation to a specific population

Morgue: The location where the bodies of deceased persons are kept until identified and claimed or are released for burial

Morphology: The science of structure and form of organisms without regard to function

Morphology axis: Structural change in tissue

Mortality: 1. The incidence of death in a specific population 2. The loss of subjects during the course of a clinical research study; *Also called* **attrition**

Mortality rate: A rate that measures the risk of death for the cause under study in a defined population during a given time period

Mortality review: A review of deaths as part of an analysis of ongoing outcome and performance improvement

Mortgage: A loan that is secured by a long-term asset, usually real estate

Most significant diagnosis: *See* **principal diagnosis**

Motion for summary judgment: A request made by the defendant in a civil case to have the case ruled in his or her favor based on the assertion that the plaintiff has no genuine issue to be tried

Motion video: A medium for storing, manipulating, and displaying moving images in a format, such as frames, that can be presented on a computer monitor; *Also called* **frame data**; **streaming video**

Motivation: The drive to accomplish a task

Motor: Related to movement of muscles and coordination; includes both large motor skills, such as walking, and fine motor skills, such as buttoning and zipping clothing

Movement diagram: A chart depicting the location of furniture and equipment in a work area and showing the usual flow of individuals or materials as they progress through the work area

MP: *See* **malpractice**

MPFS: Medicare physician fee schedule

MPFSDB: Medicare Provider Fee Schedule Data Base

MPI: *See* **master patient index; master population index**

MRI: *See* **magnetic resonance image**

MSA: *See* **metropolitan statistical area**

MSA plans: *See* **medical savings account plans**

MSDS: *See* **material safety data sheet**

MSN: *See* **Medicare summary notice**

MSO: *See* **management service organization**

MSP: *See* **Medicare secondary payer**

M technology: An operating system developed more than 25 years ago and still widely used today, which uses "write once, run anywhere" characteristics; formerly Massachusetts General Hospital Utility Multiprogramming System (MUMPS)

MUEs: *See* **Medically Unlikely Edits**

MUGA: Multiple gated acquisition scan; noninvasive test about heart muscle activity

Multi-axial: The ability of a nomenclature to express the meaning of a concept across several axes

Multi-axial system: A system that can classify an entity in several different ways

Multidimensional analysis: Simultaneous analysis of data from multiple dimensions using different data elements

Multidimensional database management system (MDDBMS): A database management system specifically designed to handle data organized into a data structure with numerous dimensions

Multidimensional data structure: A structure whereby data are organized according to the dimensions associated with them

Multidimensional online analytical processing (MOLAP): A data access methodology that is coupled tightly with a multidimensional database management system to allow the user to perform business analyses

Multidisciplinary care pathways: The process of integrating each healthcare professional's standards of care to provide better treatment for each patient

Multimedia: The combination of free-text, raster or vector graphics, sound, and/or motion video or frame data

Multipurpose Internet mail extension (MIME): A standard developed for the transmission of nontextual information via e-mail

Multivariate: A term used in reference to research studies indicating that many variables were involved

Multivoting technique: A decision-making method for determining group consensus on the prioritization of issues or solutions

MUMPS: *See* **Massachusetts General Hospital Utility Multiprogramming System**

Municipal ordinance/code: A rule established by a local branch of government such as a town, city, or county

MVPS: *See* **Medicare volume performance standard**

NAACCR: *See* **North American Association of Central Cancer Registries**

NACHRI classification: *See* **National Association of Children's Hospitals and Related Institutions classification**

NAHIT: *See* **National Alliance for Health Information Technology**

NAHQ: *See* **National Association of Healthcare Quality**

NANDA II: *See* **North American Nursing Diagnosis Association International Taxonomy**

NAR: *See* **nursing assessment record**

National Alliance for Health Information Technology (NAHIT): A partnership of government and private sector leaders from various healthcare organizations that worked toward using technology to achieve improvements in patient safety, quality of care, and operating performance; founded in 2002; ceased operations in 2009

National Association of Children's Hospitals and Related Institutions (NACHRI) classification: A classification of congenital and chronic health conditions that uses disease progression factors for case-mix analysis

National Association of Healthcare Quality (NAHQ): An organization devoted to advancing the profession of healthcare quality improvement through its accreditation program

National Cancer Institute (NCI) Thesaurus: Interoperability standard that describes anatomical locations for clinical, surgical, pathological, and research purposes of the cancer domain

National Cancer Registrars Association (NCRA): An organization of cancer registry professionals that promotes research and education in cancer registry administration and practice

National Cardiovascular Data Registry: A database supported by Medicare and maintained by the American College of Cardiologists that requires hospitals who are reimbursed by Medicare for implantable cardiac defibrillators to submit data on patients who receive implants to the registry

National Centers for Health Statistics (NCHS): The federal agency responsible for collecting and disseminating information on health services utilization and the health status of the population in the United States; developed the clinical modification to the International Classification of Diseases, Ninth Revision (ICD-9) and is responsible for updating the diagnosis portion of the ICD-9-CM

National Codes (or Level II HCPCS codes): Codes, consisting of one alpha character (A through V) followed by four digits, created by the Centers for Medicare and Medicaid Services to supplement CPT codes by describing nonphysician procedures, durable medical equipment, or specific supplies

National Commission on Correctional Health Care: An accreditation organization that maintains comprehensive standards for healthcare in correctional facilities throughout the United States

National Committee for Quality Assurance (NCQA): A private not-for-profit accreditation organization whose mission is to evaluate and report on the quality of managed care organizations in the United States

National Committee on Vital and Health Statistics (NCVHS): A public policy advisory board that recommends policy to the National Center for Health Statistics and other health-related federal programs

National conversion factor (CF): A mathematical factor used to convert relative value units into monetary payments for services provided to Medicare beneficiaries

National Correct Coding Initiative (NCCI): A series of coding regulations to prevent fraud and abuse in Medicare Part B claims; specifically addresses unbundling and mutually exclusive procedures

National Council for Prescription Drug Programs (NCPDP): A not-for-profit ANSI-accredited standards development organization founded in 1977 that develops standards for exchanging prescription and payment information

National Coverage Determination (NCD): An NCD sets forth the extent to which Medicare will cover specific services, procedures, or technologies on a national basis. Medicare contractors are required to follow NCDs

National Drug Code (NDC) Directory: A list of all drugs manufactured, prepared, propagated, compounded, or processed by a drug establishment registered under the Federal Food, Drug, and Cosmetic Act

National Drug Codes (NDC): Codes that serve as product identifiers for human drugs, currently limited to prescription drugs and a few selected over-the-counter products

National Drug File—Reference Terminology (NDF-RT): File of drug products centrally maintained and developed by the Department of Veterans Affairs that can be locally modified and deployed

National Guideline Clearinghouse (NGC): NGC is an initiative of the Agency for Healthcare Research and Quality (AHRQ), US Department of Health and Human Services. NGC was originally created by AHRQ in partnership with the American Medical Association and the American Association of Health Plans (now America's Health Insurance Plans [AHIP]); mission is to provide physicians and other health professionals, healthcare providers, health plans, integrated delivery systems, purchasers, and others an accessible mechanism for obtaining objective, detailed information on clinical practice guidelines and to further their dissemination, implementation, and use

National Health Care Survey: A national public health survey that contains data abstracted manually from a sample of acute care hospitals and discharged inpatient records, or obtained from state or other discharge databases

National health information infrastructure (NHII): An initiative set forth to improve the effectiveness, efficiency, and overall quality of health and healthcare in the United States; a comprehensive knowledge-based network of interoperable systems of clinical, public health, and personal health information that would improve decision-making by making health information available when and where it is needed; the set of technologies, standards, applications, systems, values, and laws that support all facets of individual health, healthcare, and public health

National Information Infrastructure—Health Information Network Program (NII–HIN): A national quasi-governmental organization that provides oversight of all healthcare information standards in the United States

National Institute for Standards and Technology (NIST): An agency of the US Department of Commerce, NIST was founded in 1901 as the nation's first federal physical science research laboratory

National Institutes of Health (NIH): Federal agency of the Department of Health and Human Services that is the primary agency for conducting and reporting medical research; NIH investigates the prevention, causes, and treatments for diseases

National Labor Relations Act (Wagner Act): Federal pro-union legislation that provides, among other things, procedures for union representation and prohibits unfair labor practices by unions, such as coercing nonstriking employees, and by employers, such as interference with the union selection process and discrimination against employees who support a union; passed in 1935 and later amended by the Taft-Hartley Act

National Level Repository (NLR): Data repository that manages and administers incentive payment disbursements to medical professionals, hospitals, and other organizations for applicable Medicare and Medicaid programs; a data repository for processing payment transactions for healthcare professionals, agencies and institutions for EHR incentives

National Library of Medicine (NLM): The world's largest medical library and a branch of the National Institutes of Health

National patient safety goals (NPSGs): Goals issued by the Joint Commission to improve patient safety in healthcare organizations nationwide

National Permanent Codes: These HCPCS level II codes provide a standard coding system that is managed by private and public insurers and provides a stable environment for claims submission and processing

National Practitioner Data Bank (NPDB): A data bank established by the federal government through the 1986 Health Care Quality Improvement Act that contains information on professional review actions taken against physicians and other licensed healthcare practitioners that healthcare organizations are required to verify as part of the credentialing process

National provider file (NPF): A file developed by the Centers for Medicare and Medicaid Services that includes all healthcare providers, including nonphysicians, and sites of care

National provider identifier (NPI): An eight-character alphanumeric identifier used to identify providers of healthcare services, supplies, and equipment for Medicare billing purposes

National Quality Forum: A private, not-for-profit membership organization created to develop and implement a nationwide strategy to improve the measurement and reporting of healthcare quality

National Regulatory Commission: A body that has oversight responsibility for the medical use of ionizing radiation and to which medical events must be reported

National Research Act of 1974: An act that required the Department of Health, Education, and Welfare (now the Department of Health and Human Services) to codify its policy for the protection of human subjects into federal regulations, and created a commission that generated the Belmont Report

National standard episode amount: Set dollar amount (conversion factor, constant, across-the-board multiplier), unadjusted for geographic differences, that is multiplied with the weights of the health insurance prospective payment system (HIPPS) codes in the home health prospective payment system (HHPPS). The amount for each year is published in the *Federal Register*

National standard per-visit rates: Rates for six home health disciplines based on historical claims data that are used in the payment of low-utilization payment adjustments and the calculation of outliers

National unadjusted copayment: Set dollar amount, unadjusted for geographic differences, that beneficiaries pay under the hospital outpatient prospective payment system (HOPPS)

National unadjusted payment: Product of the conversion factor multiplied by the relative weight, unadjusted for geographic differences

National Uniform Billing Committee (NUBC): The national group responsible for identifying data elements and designing the CMS-1500

National Uniform Claim Committee (NUCC): The national group that replaced the Uniform Claim Form Task Force in 1995 and developed a standard data set to be used in the transmission of noninstitutional provider claims to and from third-party payers

National Vaccine Advisory Committee (NVAC): A national advisory group that advises and makes recommendations to support the director of the National Vaccine Program

National Vital Statistics System (NVSS): The oldest and most successful example of intergovernmental data sharing in public health, and the shared relationships, standards, and procedures that form the mechanism by which NCHS collects and disseminates the nation's official vital statistics. These data are provided through contracts between NCHS and vital registration systems operated in the various jurisdictions and legally responsible for the registration of vital events—births, deaths, marriages, divorces, and fetal deaths

Nationwide Health Information Network (NHIN): A set of standards, services, and policies that enable secure health information exchange over the Internet. The network provides a foundation for the exchange of health information across diverse entities, within communities, and across the country, helping to achieve the goals of the HITECH Act

Naturalism: A philosophy of research that assumes that multiple contextual truths exist and bias is always present; *See* **qualitative approach**

Naturalistic observation: A type of nonparticipant observation in which researchers observe certain behaviors and events as they occur naturally

Natural language: A fifth-generation computer programming language that uses human language to give people a more natural connection with computers

Natural language processing (NLP): A technology that converts human language (structured or unstructured) into data that can be translated then manipulated by computer systems; branch of artificial intelligence

NB: *See* **newborn**

NCI: National Cancer Institute

NCCI: *See* **National Correct Coding Initiative**

NCD: *See* **national coverage determination**

NCHS: *See* **National Centers for Health Statistics**

NCI Thesaurus: *See* **National Cancer Institute Thesaurus**

NCPDP: *See* **National Council on Prescription Drug Programs**

NCQA: *See* **National Committee for Quality Assurance**

NCR: *See* **no carbon required**

NCRA: *See* **National Cancer Registrars Association**

NCS: nerve conduction study

NCVHS: *See* **National Committee on Vital and Health Statistics**

NDC: *See* **National Drug Codes**

NDF-RT: *See* **National Drug File—Reference Terminology**

Near miss: An opportunity to improve patient safety–related practices based on a condition or incident with potential for more serious consequences

NEC: *See* **not elsewhere classified**

Necropsy: *See* **autopsy**

Need for intervention: A term that relates to the severity-of-illness consequences that would result from the lack of immediate or continuing medical care

Needs assessment: A procedure performed by collecting and analyzing data to determine what is required, lacking, or desired by an employee, a group, or an organization

Need-to-know principle: The release-of-information principle based on the minimum necessary standard

Negative relationship: A relationship in which the effects move in opposite directions; *Also called* **inverse relationship**

Negligence: A legal term that refers to the result of an action by an individual who does not act the way a reasonably prudent person would act under the same circumstances

Neonatal death: The death of a live-born infant within the first 27 days, 23 hours, and 59 minutes following the moment of birth

Neonatal mortality rate: The number of deaths of infants under 28 days of age during a given time period divided by the total number of births for the same time period

Neonatal period: The period of an infant's life from the hour of birth through the first 27 days, 23 hours, and 59 minutes of life

Net: A term used in financial management to refer to the value of something, incorporating both the historical cost and anything that adds to or detracts from that value

Net assets: The organization's resources remaining after subtracting its liabilities

Net autopsy rate: The ratio of inpatient autopsies compared to inpatient deaths calculated by dividing the total number of inpatient autopsies performed by the hospital pathologist for a given time period by the total number of inpatient deaths minus unautopsied coroners' or medical examiners' cases for the same time period

Net death rate: The total number of inpatient deaths minus the number of deaths that occurred less than 48 hours after admission for a given time period divided by the total number of inpatient discharges minus the number of deaths that occurred less than 48 hours after admission for the same time period

Net income: The difference between total revenues and total expenses; *See* **profit**

Net loss: The condition when total expenses exceed total revenue

Net present value (NPV): A formula used to assess the current value of a project when the monies used were invested in the organization's investment vehicles rather than expended for the project; this value is then compared to the allocation of the monies and the cash inflows of the project, both of which are adjusted to current time

Net value: The purchase price of an item less its depreciation

Network: 1. A type of information technology that connects different computers and computer systems so they can share information 2. Physicians, hospitals, and other providers who provide healthcare services to members of a managed care organization; providers may be associated through formal or informal contracts and agreements

Network administrators: The individuals involved in installing, configuring, managing, monitoring, securing, and maintaining network computer applications and responsible for supporting the network infrastructure and controlling user access

Network computer: A personal computer with a computer processing unit but no storage; a type of computer that is used to run applications on servers over a network rather than from the hard disk of the computer, and all data is stored on the server; *Also called* **thin client**

Network control: A method of protecting data from unauthorized change and corruption at rest and during transmission among information systems

Networking: The use of specific technology, including items such as bridges and routers, to connect disparate systems so they may share information

Network model: Type of health maintenance organization (HMO) in which the HMO contracts with two or more medical groups and reimburses the groups on a fee-for-service or capitation basis; *See* **group practice model**

Network model health maintenance program: Program in which participating HMOs contract for services with one or more multispecialty group practices; *See* **network model**

Network protocol: A set of conventions that governs the exchange of data between hardware and/or software components in a communications network

Network provider: A physician or another healthcare professional who is a member of a managed care network

Neural networks: Nonlinear predictive models that, using a set of data that describe what a person wants to find, detect a pattern to match a particular profile through a training process involving interactive learning

Neutral zone: Bridges's transitional stage in organizational change in which the past has been left but the future stage is not yet clearly established

New beginnings: Bridges's final stage of transition management in which the new organization is formed

New patient: An individual who has not received professional services from the physician, or any other physician of the same specialty in the same practice group before or within a designated time frame; an individual who has not received professional services from any provider of a organization/healthcare facility before or within a designated time frame

Newborn (NB): An inpatient who was born in a hospital at the beginning of the current inpatient hospitalization

Newborn autopsy rate: The number of autopsies performed on newborns who died during a given time period divided by the total number of newborns who died during the same time period

Newborn bassinet count: The number of available hospital newborn bassinets, both occupied and vacant, on any given day

Newborn bassinet count day: A unit of measure that denotes the presence of one newborn bassinet, either occupied or vacant, set up and staffed for use in one 24-hour period

Newborn death rate: The number of newborns who died divided by the total number of newborns, both alive and dead; *Also called* newborn mortality rate

NGC: *See* **National Guideline Clearinghouse**

NHII: *See* **national health information infrastructure**

NIC: *See* **Nursing Interventions Classification**

NIDSEC: *See* **Nursing Information and Data Set Evaluation Center**

NIH: *See* **National Institutes of Health**

NII-HIN: *See* **National Information Infrastructure—Health Information Network Program**

NIST: *See* **National Institute for Standards and Technology**

NLM: *See* **National Library of Medicine**

NLP: *See* **natural language processing**

NLR: *See* **National Level Repository**

NMDS: *See* **Nursing Minimum Data Set**

NMJ: neuromuscular junction studies

NMMDS: *See* **Nursing Management Minimum Data Set**

NOC: *See* **Nursing Outcomes Classification**

No man's land: The zone in the palmar or volar surface of the hand between the distal palmar crease (the crease in the palm closest to the fingers) and the middle of the middle phalanx (middle finger)

Nomenclature: A recognized system of terms used in a science or art that follows preestablished naming conventions; a disease nomenclature is a listing of the proper name for each disease entity with its specific code number

Nominal data: A type of data that represents values or observations that can be labeled or named and where the values fall into unordered categories; *Also called* **dichotomous data**; *See* **nominal-level data**

Nominal group technique: A group process technique that involves the steps of silent listing, recording each participant's list, discussing, and rank ordering the priority or importance of items; allows groups to narrow the focus of discussion or to make decisions without becoming involved in extended, circular discussions

Nominal-level data: Data that fall into groups or categories that are mutually exclusive and with no specific order (for example, patient demographics such as third-party payer, race, and sex); *Also called* **categorical data**

Noncovered procedures: Services not reimbursable under a managed care plan

Nondisclosure agreement: An agreement relating to the confidentiality and privacy of patient information employees may be required to sign as a condition of employment

Nonexempt employees: All groups of employees covered by the provisions of the Fair Labor Standards Act

Nonfeasance: A type of negligence meaning failure to act

Nonlabor share (portion, ratio): Facilities' operating costs not related to labor (typically 25 to 30 percent); *See* **labor-related share**

Nonlicensed practitioner: A healthcare worker who does not hold a public license or certification and who is supervised by a licensed or certified healthcare professional in delivering care to patients

Nonmaleficence: A legal principle that means "first do no harm"

Nonoperating room procedure: A type of procedure that is considered in assigning a diagnosis-related group but usually does not require the use of an operating room

Nonparametric technique: A type of statistical procedure used for variables that are not normally distributed in a population; *See* **distribution-free technique**

NonPARs: *See* **nonparticipating physicians**; **nonparticipating provider**

Nonparticipant observation: A method of research in which researchers act as neutral observers who do not intentionally interact or affect the actions of the population being observed

Nonparticipating physicians (nonPARs): Physicians who treat Medicare beneficiaries but do not have a legal agreement with the program to accept assignment on all Medicare services and who, therefore, may bill beneficiaries more than the Medicare reasonable charge on a service-by-service basis

Nonparticipating provider: A healthcare provider who did not sign a participation agreement with Medicare and so is not obligated to accept assignment on Medicare claims

Nonprogrammed decision: A decision that involves careful and deliberate thought and discussion because of a unique, complex, or changing situation

Nonrandom sampling: A type of convenience or purposive sampling in which all members of the target population do not have an equal or independent chance of being selected for a research study

Nonrepudiation: The claim which guarantees that the source of the health record documentation cannot deny later that he or she was the author

Nonroutine medical supplies: Supplies that are furnished either directly or under an arrangement with an outside supplier in which a home health agency, rather than the supplier, bills Medicare and the agency pays the supplier

Nonselective catheter placement: Catheter placement into the aorta, vena cava, or the vessel punctured

No-RAP (request for anticipated payment) low-utilization payment adjustment: A type of claim submitted for an episode when the home health agency is aware from the outset that the episode will require no more than four visits

Normal distribution: A theoretical family of continuous frequency distributions characterized by a symmetric bell-shaped curve, with an equal mean, median, and mode; any standard deviation; and with half of the observations above the mean and half below it

Normalization: 1. A formal process applied to relational database design to determine which variables should be grouped together in a table in order to reduce data redundancy across and within the table 2. Conversion of various representational forms to standard expressions so those that have the same meaning will be recognized by computer software as synonymous in a data search

Normative decision model: A decision tree developed by Vroom-Yetton to determine when to make decisions independently or collaboratively or by delegation

Norming: The third of the four steps in forming a functional team, during which each team member comes to understand his or her role

North American Association of Central Cancer Registries (NAACCR): A national organization that certifies state, population-based cancer registries

North American Nursing Diagnosis Association International Taxonomy (NANDA II): Nursing terminology used to develop and classify nursing diagnoses in a taxonomy

NOS: *See* **not otherwise specified**

Nosocomial infection: An infection acquired by a patient while receiving care or services in a healthcare organization; *See* **hospital-acquired infection**

Nosocomial infection rate: The number of hospital-acquired infections for a given time period divided by the total number of inpatient discharges for the same time period

Nosology: The branch of medical science that deals with classification systems

Not elsewhere classified (NEC): A type of classification that indicates that there is no separate code for the condition even though the diagnostic statement is specific

Not otherwise specified (NOS): A type of classification that denotes a lack of information in the record and means unspecified rather than not elsewhere classified

Not-for-profit organization: An organization that is not owned by individuals whose profits are retained by the organization and reinvested back into the organization for the benefit of the community it serves

Notice of privacy practices: A statement (mandated by the HIPAA Privacy Rule) issued by a healthcare organization that informs individuals of the uses and disclosures of patient-identifiable health information that may be made by the organization, as well as the individual's rights and the organization's legal duties with respect to that information

Notice of Proposed Rulemaking (NPRM): Notice published in the *Federal Register* calling for public comment on its policy; the public at large has a specified time period to submit comments

Notifiable disease: A disease that must be reported to a government agency so that regular, frequent, and timely information on individual cases can be used to prevent and control future cases of the disease

NP: *See* **nurse practitioner**

NPDB: *See* **National Practitioner Data Bank**

NPF: *See* **national provider file**
NPI: *See* **national provider identifier**
NPRM: *See* **Notice of Proposed Rulemaking**
NPSGs: *See* **national patient safety goals**
NPV: *See* **net present value**
NUBC: *See* **National Uniform Billing Committee**
NUCC: *See* **National Uniform Claim Committee**
Nuclear medicine: A method of examination in which technologists using a special camera introduce radioactive substances into the body orally, intravenously, or by ventilated aerosol or gas. A special camera is used to detect the radioactive substances as they circulate through the body and produce an image
Null hypothesis: A hypothesis that states there is no association between the independent and dependent variables in a research study
Numerator: The part of a fraction that is above the line and signifies the number of parts of the denominator taken
Numerical data: Data that include discrete data and continuous data
Numeric filing system: A system of health record identification and storage in which records are arranged consecutively in ascending numerical order according to the health record number
Nurse practitioner (NP): A registered nurse (RN) with advanced training authorized to provide basic primary healthcare, diagnosing and treating common acute illnesses and injuries, including prescribing medications
Nursing assessment: The assessment performed by a nurse to obtain clinical and personal information about a patient shortly after he or she has been admitted to a nursing unit
Nursing assessment record (NAR): A form used to track patients' functional status; supports the Minimum Data Set (MDS) process; *Also called* activities of daily living (ADL) flow sheet
Nursing facility: A comprehensive term for long-term care facilities that provide nursing care and related services on a 24-hour basis for residents requiring medical, nursing, or rehabilitative care
Nursing Home Quality Initiative: A six-state pilot project performed in 2002 by the Centers for Medicare and Medicaid Services (CMS) that identifies quality

measures that reflect the quality of care in nursing homes

Nursing Home Reform Act: A part of the Omnibus Budget Reconciliation Act of 1987 whose purpose is to guarantee the quality of nursing home care and to ensure that the care that residents receive helps them to achieve or maintain the "highest practicable" level of physical, mental, and psychosocial well-being

Nursing informatics: The field of information science concerned with the management of data and information used to support the practice and delivery of nursing care through the application of computers and computer technologies

Nursing Information and Data Set Evaluation Center (NIDSEC): The Nursing Information and Data Set Evaluation Center was established by the American Nurses Association (ANA) to review, evaluate against defined criteria, and recognize information systems from developers and manufacturers that support documentation of nursing care within automated nursing information systems (NIS) or within computer-based patient record systems (CPR)

Nursing information system (NIS): Information system that assists in the planning and monitoring of overall patient care and documents the nursing care provided to a patient

Nursing Interventions Classification (NIC): A terminology that describes the treatments that nurses perform

Nursing Management Minimum Data Set (NMMDS): A data set that supports description, analysis, and comparisons of nursing care and nursing resources in the context of complex healthcare outcomes; designed to complement the clinical patient-oriented data designated in the nursing minimum data set (NMDS)

Nursing Minimum Data Set (NMDS): A data set that provides uniform definitions and categories of nursing care; built on the uniform minimum health data sets (UMHDS)

Nursing notes: Health record documentation that describes the nursing staff's observations of the patient and records the clinical and therapeutic services provided to the patient as well as the patient's response to treatment

Nursing Outcomes Classification (NOC): A classification of patient or client outcomes developed to evaluate the effects of nursing interventions

Nursing vocabulary: A classification system used to capture documentation on nursing care

Nutritional assessment: The assessment performed by a registered dietitian to obtain information about a patient's diet history, weight and height, appetite and food preferences, and food sensitivities and allergies

NVAC: *See* **National Vaccine Advisory Committee**

NVSS: *See* **National Vital Statistics System**

OASIS: *See* **Outcomes and Assessment Information Set**

OB: Obstetrics

OB/GYN: Obstetrics and gynecology

Object: The basic component in an object-oriented database that includes both data and their relationships within a single structure

Objective: A statement of the end result expected, stated in measurable terms, usually with a time limitation (deadline date) and often with a cost estimate or limitation

Objectivity: An accounting concept in which assets are classified at historical cost or current value

Object-oriented database (OODB): A type of database that uses commands that act as small, self-contained instructional units (objects) that may be combined in various ways

Object-oriented database management system (OODBMS): A specific set of software programs used to implement an object-oriented database

Object-oriented framework: A new way of programming and representing data that uses commands that act as small, self-contained instructional units that may be combined in various ways to produce larger programs

Object-relational database: A type of database (both object-oriented and relational) that stores both objects and traditional tables

Object request broker (ORB): The messenger at the heart of the object-oriented framework that acts as a relay station between client and server

OBRA of 1987: *See* **Omnibus Budget Reconciliation Act of 1987**

OBRA of 1989: *See* **Omnibus Budget Reconciliation Act of 1989**

Observation: Service in which providers observe and monitor a patient to decide whether the patient needs to be admitted to inpatient care or can be discharged to home or an outpatient area, usually charged by the hour

Observational research: A method of research in which researchers obtain data by watching research participants rather than by asking questions

Observational study: An epidemiological study in which the exposure and outcome for each individual in the study is observed

Observation patient: A patient who presents with a medical condition with a significant degree of instability and disability and who needs to be monitored, evaluated, and assessed to determine whether he or she should be admitted for inpatient care or discharged for care in another setting

Occasion of service: A specified identifiable service involved in the care of a patient that is not an encounter (for example, a lab test ordered during an encounter)

Occlusion: Completely closing an orifice or the lumen of a tubular body part

Occupancy percent/ratio: *See* **bed occupancy ratio**

Occupation: The employment, business, or course of action in which the patient is engaged

Occupational health: The degree to which an employee is able to function at an optimum level of well-being at work as reflected by productivity, work attendance, disability compensation claims, and employment longevity

Occupational health services: Health services involving the physical, mental, and social well-being of individuals in relation to their work and working environment

Occupational Safety and Health Act (OSHA) of 1970: The federal legislation that established comprehensive safety and health guidelines for employers

Occupational Safety and Health Administration (OSHA): Ensures safe and healthful working conditions for working men and women by setting and enforcing standards and by providing training, outreach, education, and assistance

Occupational safety and health record: A record kept on an employee as part of employment that contains any and all information related to such items as medical tests, drug tests, examinations, physical abilities, immunizations, screenings required by law, biohazardous exposure, and physical limitations; OSHA regulations ensure that an employee (or designated representative) is given access to his or her own medical and exposure records within 15 days of request

Occupational therapy (OT): A treatment that uses constructive activities to help restore the resident's ability to carry out needed activities of daily living and improves or maintains functional ability

Occurrence report: A structured data collection tool that risk managers use to gather information about potentially compensable events; *Also called* **incident report**

Occurrence screening: A risk management technique in which the risk manager reviews the health records of current and discharged hospital inpatients with the goal of identifying potentially compensable events; *Also called* **generic screening**

OCE: *See* **outpatient code editor**

OCR technology: *See* **optical character recognition technology**

OD: *See* **organizational development**

Odds ratio: A relative measure of occurrence of an illness; the odds of exposure in a diseased group divided by the odds of exposure in a nondiseased group

OER: *See* **outcomes and effectiveness research**

Office for Civil Rights (OCR): Department in HHS responsible for enforcing civil rights laws that prohibit discrimination on the basis of race, color, national origin, disability, age, sex, and religion by healthcare and human services entities over which OCR has jurisdiction, such as state and local social and health services agencies, and hospitals, clinics, nursing homes, or other entities receiving federal financial assistance from HHS. This office also has the authority to ensure and enforce the HIPAA Privacy and Security Rules; OCR is responsible for investigating all alleged violations of the Privacy and Security Rules

Office for Human Research Protections (OHRP): Provides leadership in the protection of the rights, welfare, and well-being of subjects involved in research conducted or supported by the US Department of Health and Human Services (HHS). OHRP helps ensure this by providing clarification and guidance, developing educational programs and materials, maintaining regulatory oversight, and providing advice on ethical and regulatory issues in biomedical and social-behavioral research

Office of Management and Budget (OMB): The core mission of OMB is to serve the President of the United States in implementing his vision across the Executive Branch. OMB is the largest component of the Executive Office of the President. It reports directly to the President and helps a wide range of executive departments and agencies across the federal government to implement the commitments and priorities of the President

Office of Research Integrity (ORI): Promotes integrity in biomedical and behavioral research supported by the US Public Health Service (PHS) at about 4,000 institutions worldwide. ORI monitors institutional investigations of research misconduct and facilitates the responsible conduct of research (RCR) through educational, preventive, and regulatory activities

Office of the Inspector General (OIG): Mandated by Public Law 95-452 (as amended) to protect the integrity of Department of Health and Human Services (HHS) programs, as well as the health and welfare of the beneficiaries of those programs. The OIG has a responsibility to report both to the Secretary and to the Congress program and management problems and recommendations to correct them. The OIG's duties are carried out through a nationwide network of audits, investigations, inspections, and other mission-related functions performed by OIG components

Office of the Inspector General (OIG) Workplan: Yearly plan released by the OIG that outlines the focus for reviews and investigations in various healthcare settings

Office of the National Coordinator for Health Information Technology (ONC): The principal federal entity charged with coordination of nationwide efforts to implement and use the most advanced health information technology and the electronic exchange of health information. The position of National Coordinator was created in 2004, through an Executive Order, and legislatively mandated in the Health Information Technology for Economic and Clinical Health Act (HITECH Act) of 2009

Offshoring: Outsourcing jobs to countries overseas, wherein local employees abroad perform jobs that domestic employees previously performed

OHCA: *See* **Organized Healthcare Arrangement**

OIG: *See* **Office of the Inspector General**

OLAP: *See* **online analytical processing**

OLTP: *See* **online transaction processing**

Omaha System: A research-based taxonomy designed to generate data following routine client care

Omnibus Budget Reconciliation Act (OBRA) of 1987: Federal legislation passed in 1987 that required the Health Care Financing Administration (now renamed the Centers for Medicare and Medicaid Services) to develop an assessment instrument (called the resident assessment instrument) to standardize the collection of patient data from skilled nursing facilities

Omnibus Budget Reconciliation Act (OBRA) of 1989: The federal legislation that mandated important changes in the payment rules for Medicare physicians; specifically, the legislation that requires nursing facilities to conduct regular patient assessments for Medicare and Medicaid beneficiaries

OMT: Osteopathic manipulative treatment

ONC: *See* **Office of the National Coordinator for Health Information Technology**

One-tailed hypothesis: An alternative hypothesis in which the researcher makes a prediction in one direction

One-to-many relationship: A relationship that exists when one instance of an entity is associated with multiple instances of another entity

One-to-one relationship: A relationship that exists when an instance of an entity is associated with only one instance of another entity, and vice versa

Ongoing records review: *See* **open-record review**

Online analytical processing (OLAP): A data access architecture that allows the user to retrieve specific information from a large volume of data; *See* **online transaction processing**

Online analytical processing (OLAP) engine: An optimized query generator that can retrieve the correct information from the warehouse to accommodate what-if queries

Online/real-time analytical processing (OLAP): *See* **online analytical processing**

Online/real-time transaction processing (OLTP): The real-time processing of day-to-day business transactions from a database; *See* **online analytical processing**

On-the-job training: A method of training in which an employee learns necessary skills and processes by performing the functions of his or her position

Ontology: A common vocabulary organized by meaning, allowing for an understanding of the structure of descriptive information that facilitates a specific topic or domain

OODB: *See* **object-oriented database**

OODBMS: *See* **object-oriented database management system**

Open-ended HMO: *See* **point-of-service (POS) plan**

Open-ended question: *See* **unstructured question**

Opening conference: A meeting conducted at the beginning of the Joint Commission accreditation site visit during which the surveyors outline the schedule of activities and list any individuals whom they would like to interview

Open record: The health record of a patient who is still receiving services in the facility

Open-record review: A review of the health records of patients currently in the hospital or under active treatment; part of the Joint Commission survey process

Open records laws: Laws that define what information is subject to public disclosure and are used to deny FOIA requests that include PHI; *Also called* freedom of information laws; public records

Open system: A system which permits other parties to produce products that interoperate with it; a computer is an open system

Operating budget: The budget that summarizes the anticipated expenses for a department's routine, day-to-day operations

Operating clinician identification: The unique national identification number assigned to the clinician who performed the principal procedure

Operating room (OR): The area in a healthcare facility that is equipped and staffed to provide facilities and personnel for the performance of surgical procedures

Operating room (OR) procedure: Procedure that the physician panel classifies as occurring in the operating room in most hospitals; presence of an OR procedure groups a case to a surgical diagnosis-related group (DRG)

Operating system: The principal piece of software in any computer system, which consists of a master set of programs that manage the basic operations of the computer

Operation: *See* **surgical operation**

Operational budget: A type of budget that allocates and controls resources to meet an organization's goals and objectives for the fiscal year

Operational decision making: A process for addressing problems that come up in the day-to-day operation of a business unit or the day-to-day execution of a work task

Operational plan: The short-term objectives set by an organization to improve its methods of doing business and achieve its planned outcomes

Operation index: A list of the operations and surgical procedures performed in a healthcare facility, which is sequenced according to the code numbers of the classification system in use

Operation Restore Trust: A 1995 joint effort of the Department of Health and Human Services (HHS), Office of the Inspector General (OIG), the Centers for Medicare and Medicaid Services (CMS), and the Administration of Aging (AOA) to target fraud and abuse among healthcare providers

Operations analysis: *See* **workflow analysis**

Operations management: The application of mathematical and statistical techniques to production and distribution efficiency

Operations research (OR): A scientific discipline primarily begun around the World War II era that seeks to apply the scientific method and mathematical models to the solution of a variety of management decision problems

Operations support systems (OSS): An information system that facilitates the operational management of a healthcare organization such as telecommunications or bed boards and patient flow; varies by organization

Operative report: A formal document that describes the events surrounding a surgical procedure or operation and identifies the principal participants in the surgery

Opportunity for improvement: A healthcare structure, product, service, process, or outcome that does not meet its customers' expectations and, therefore, could be improved

OPPS: *See* **outpatient prospective payment system**

Optical character recognition (OCR) technology: A method of encoding text from analog paper into bitmapped images and translating the images into a form that is computer readable

Optical image-based system: A health record system in which information is created initially in paper form and then scanned into an electronic system for storage and retrieval

Optical imaging technology: The process by which information is scanned onto optical disks

Optimization (as related to clinical coding): The process of thoroughly reviewing the health record to identify all procedures performed and services rendered by the physician to ensure accurate and complete coding for optimum reimbursement

Opt-in/Opt-out: A type of HIE model that sets the default for health information of patients to be included automatically, but the patient can opt out completely

Opt-in with restrictions: A type of HIE model in which the default is set where no patient health information is automatically made available; patients must define what information is to be sent, who it is sent to, and for what purposes the information may be used

Opt-out with exceptions: Sets the defaults for health information of patients to be included, but the patient can opt out completely or allow only select data to be included

OR: *See* **operating room** or **operations research**

OR procedure: *See* **operating room procedure**

Orange book: The common name for the US Department of Defense document that defines the trusted computer system evaluation criteria, from which many of the security criteria for healthcare systems are being drawn

ORB: *See* **object request broker**

Order entry: The use of a computer and decision support to record and initiate the transmission of a physician's order

Orders for restraint or seclusion: Physician's orders for physical or pharmaceutical restraint or seclusion to protect the patient or others from harm

Ordinal data: A type of data that represents values or observations that can be ranked or ordered; *See* **ordinal-level data**

Ordinal-level data: Data with inherent order and with higher numbers usually associated with higher values; *Also called* **ordinal data; ranked data**

Ordinal scale of measurement: Measurement scale that consists of separate categories with separate names ranked in terms of magnitude

Organization: The planned coordination of the activities for more than one person for the achievement of a common purpose or goal

Organizational chart: A graphic representation of an organization's formal reporting structure

Organizational development (OD): The application of behavioral science research and practices to planned organizational change

Organizational lifeline: A line drawing of important historical events in the life of an organization; used for organizational development intervention reflecting on historical trends

Organizational pull model: A model in which the organization views information systems technology as the means to enable people in the organization to work more efficiently and effectively

Organized Healthcare Arrangement (OHCA): An agreement characterized by more than one covered entity who share PHI to manage and benefit their common enterprise and are recognized by the public as a single entity

Organizing: The process of coordinating something, such as activities

Orientation: A set of activities designed to familiarize new employees with their jobs, the organization, and its work culture

Orion Project: The Joint Commission's initiative designed to assess accreditation models, develop a continuous accreditation process, and test alternative processes for reporting survey findings to hospitals

ORT: Operation Restore Trust

ORYX: *See* **ORYX initiative**

ORYX initiative: The Joint Commission's initiative that supports the integration of outcomes data and other performance measurement data into the accreditation process; often referred to as ORYX

OSHA: *See* **Occupational Safety and Health Administration**

OSHA of 1970: *See* **Occupational Safety and Health Act of 1970**

OSS: *See* **operations support system**

Osteopath: A physician licensed to practice in osteopathy (a system of medical practice that is based on the manipulation of body parts as well as other therapies)

OT: *See* **occupational therapy; outlier threshold**

Other diagnoses: All conditions (recorded to the highest documented level of specificity) that coexist at the time of admission, develop subsequently, or affect the treatment received and/or length of stay

Other urban area: An urban area with a population of one million residents or fewer

Outcome: 1. The end result of healthcare treatment, which may be positive and appropriate or negative and diminishing 2. The performance (or nonperformance) of one or more processes, services, or activities by healthcare providers

Outcome indicator: A measurement of the end results of a clinical process (for example, complications, adverse effects, patient satisfaction) for an individual patient or a group of patients within a specific diagnostic category; *See* **outcome measures**

Outcome measures: 1. The process of systematically tracking a patient's clinical treatment and responses to that treatment, including measures of morbidity and functional status, for the purpose of improving care 2. A measure that indicates the result of the performance (or nonperformance) of a function or process

Outcomes analysis: *See* **outcomes assessment**

Outcomes and Assessment Information Set (OASIS): A standard core assessment data tool developed to measure the outcomes of adult patients receiving home health services under the Medicare and Medicaid programs

Outcomes and effectiveness research (OER): A type of research performed to explain the end results of specific healthcare practices and interventions

Outcomes assessment: An evaluation that measures the actual outcomes of patient care and service against predetermined criteria (expected outcomes), based on the premise that care is delivered in order to bring about certain results; *Also called* **outcomes analysis**

Outcomes management: The process of systematically tracking a patient's clinical treatment and responses to that treatment, including measures of morbidity and functional status, for the purpose of improving care; *Also called* **outcomes measurement**

Outcomes measurement: *See* **outcomes management**

Outcomes monitoring: *See* **outcomes management**

Outguide: A device used in paper-based health record systems to track the location of records removed from the file storage area

Outlier: 1. A case in a prospective payment system with unusually long lengths of stay or exceptionally high costs (day outlier or cost outlier, respectively) 2. An extreme statistical value that falls outside the normal range

Outlier payment: A payment made in addition to a full-episode payment when the cost of the services exceeds a fixed-loss threshold in the Medicare acute care prospective payment system

Outlier threshold (OT): The upper range (threshold) in length of stay before the case becomes a day outlier

Out-of-pocket: Payment made by the policyholder or member

Out-of-pocket expenses: Healthcare costs paid by the insured (for example, deductibles, copayments, and coinsurance) after which the insurer pays a percentage (often 80 or 100 percent) of covered expenses

Outpatient: A patient who receives ambulatory care services in a hospital-based clinic or department

Outpatient code editor (OCE): A software program linked to the Correct Coding Initiative that applies a set of logical rules to determine whether various combinations of codes are correct and appropriately represent the services provided; *See* **editor**

Outpatient coder: An individual responsible for assigning ICD-9-CM and CPT/HCPCS codes to ambulatory surgery, emergency department cases, or outpatient ancillary clinic visits

Outpatient prospective payment system (OPPS): The Medicare prospective payment system used for hospital-based outpatient services and procedures that is predicated on the assignment of ambulatory payment classifications

Outpatient Service Mix Index (SMI): The sum of the weights of ambulatory payment classification groups for patients treated during a given period divided by the total volume of patients treated

Outpatient unit: A hospital-based ambulatory care facility organized into sections (clinics) whose number depends on the size and degree of departmentalization of the medical or clinic staff, available facilities, type of service needed in the community, and the needs of the patients for whom it accepts responsibility

Outpatient visit: A patient's visit to one or more units located in the ambulatory services area (clinic or physician's office) of an acute care hospital in which an overnight stay does not occur

Outputs: The outcomes of inputs into a system (for example, the output of the admitting process is the patient's admission to the hospital)

Outsourcing: The hiring of an individual or a company external to an organization to perform a function either on site or off site

Outsourcing firm: A company that enters into a contract with a healthcare organization to perform services such as clinical coding or transcription

Overcoding: The practice of assigning more codes than needed to describe a patient's condition. Some instances of overcoding may be contrary to the guidance provided in the Official Coding Guidelines

Overhead costs: The expenses associated with supporting but not providing patient care services

Overlap: Situation in which a patient is issued more than one medical record number from an organization with multiple facilities

Overlay: Situation in which a patient is issued a medical record number that has been previously issued to a different patient

Owner's equity: The value of the investment in an organization by its owners

P4P: *See* **pay for performance**

P4Q: *See* **pay for quality**

PA: *See* **physician assistant**

PACE: *See* **Programs of All-Inclusive Care for the Elderly**

Package Code: The part of the National Drug Code that identifies package size

Packaging: A payment under the Medicare outpatient prospective payment system that includes items such as anesthesia, supplies, certain drugs, and the use of recovery and observation rooms

Packet switching: An information transmission system in which data are encoded into short units (packets) and sent through an electronic communications network

PACS: *See* **picture archiving and communication system**

PAI: *See* **patient assessment instrument**

Palliative care: A type of medical care designed to relieve the patient's pain and suffering without attempting to cure the underlying disease

P and T committee: *See* **P/T Committee**

Panel interview: An interview format in which the applicant is interviewed by several interviewers at the same time

Paradigm: A philosophical or theoretical framework within which a discipline formulates its theories and makes generalizations

Parallel work division: A type of concurrent work design in which one employee does several tasks and takes the job from beginning to end

Parametric technique: A type of statistical procedure that is based on the assumption that a variable is normally distributed in a population

Pareto chart: A bar graph that includes bars arranged in order of descending size to show decisions on the prioritization of issues, problems, or solutions

Par level: The accepted, standard inventory level for all supplies and equipment in an organization

PARs: *See* **participating physicians**; also, participating providers

Partial episode payment (PEP) adjustment: A reduced episode payment that may be based on the number of service days in an episode

Partial hospitalization: A limited patient stay in the hospital setting, typically as part of a transitional program to a less intense level of service; for example, psychiatric and drug and alcohol treatment facilities that offer services to help patients reenter the community, return to work, and assume family responsibilities

Partial mastectomy: The partial removal of breast tissue, leaving the breast nearly intact; sometimes called a lumpectomy

Participant observation: A research method in which researchers also participate in the observed actions

Participating physicians (PARs): Physicians who sign an agreement with Medicare to accept assignment for all services provided to Medicare beneficiaries for the duration of the agreement

Partnership: The business venture of two or more owners for whom the profits represent the owners' personal income

Part-time employee: An employee who works less than the full-time standard of 40 hours per week, 80 hours per two-week period, or 8 hours per day

PASARR: *See* **Preadmission Screening Assessment and Annual Resident Review**

Pass-through: Exception to the Medicare prospective payment systems (PPSs) for a high-cost service. The exception minimizes the negative financial impact of the lump-sum payments of the PPSs. Pass-throughs are not included in the PPSs and are passed through to cost-based (retrospective) payment mechanisms. In the hospital outpatient prospective payment system (HOPPS), the CMS created exceptions for some expensive drugs, pharmaceuticals, biologicals, and devices. Rather than being bundled or packaged, these exceptions to the CMS's HOPPS are "passed through" the HOPPS to other payment mechanisms (payment status indicators F, G, H, and J). The inpatient prospective payment system (IPPS) passes through the costs of medical education and organ acquisition and some capital costs

Password: A series of characters that must be entered to authenticate user identity and gain access to a computer or specified portions of a database

Password crackers: Software programs used to identify an unknown or forgotten password

Past, family, and/or social history (PFSH): The patient's past experience with illnesses, hospitalizations, operations, injuries, and treatments; a review of medical events in the patient's family, including diseases that may be hereditary or place the patient at risk; age-appropriate review of past and current activities

Path–goal theory: A situational leadership theory that emphasizes the role of the leader in removing barriers to goal achievement

Pathology report: A type of health record or documentation that describes the results of a microscopic and macroscopic evaluation of a specimen removed or expelled during a surgical procedure

Patient: A living or deceased individual who is receiving or has received healthcare services

Patient account number: A number assigned by a healthcare facility for billing purposes that is unique to a particular episode of care; a new account number is assigned each time the patient receives care or services at the facility

Patient advocacy: The function performed by patient representatives (sometimes called ombudsmen) who respond personally to complaints from patients and/or their families

Patient assessment instrument (PAI): A standardized tool used to evaluate the patient's condition after admission to, and at discharge from, the healthcare facility

Patient care charting system: A system in which caregivers enter data into health records

Patient Care Data Set (PCDS): A terminology of patient problems, patient care goals, and patient care orders that represents and captures clinical data for inclusion in patient care information systems

Patient care system: A type of information system that has traditionally been designed for nursing documentation

Patient care unit (PCU): An organizational entity of a healthcare facility organized both physically and functionally to provide care

Patient-Centered Medical Home (PCMH): *See* **Medical Home**

Patient day: *See* **inpatient service day**

Patient health outcome: *See* **outcome**

Patient health record: *See* **health record**

Patient history questionnaire: A series of structured questions to be answered by patients to provide information to clinicians about their past and current health status; *See* **adult health questionnaire**

Patient-identifiable data: Personal information that can be linked to a specific patient, such as age, gender, date of birth, and address

Patient medical record information (PMRI): Information in which SNOMED CT is part of a core set of terminology

Patient/member web portals: The media for providing patient or member access to the provider organization's multiple sources of data from any network-connected device

Patient monitoring system: Type of system that automatically collects and stores patient data from other various systems used in healthcare such as fetal monitoring, vital signs, and oxygen saturation rates

Patient Protection and Affordable Care Act (PPACA): A federal statute that was signed into law on March 23, 2010. Along with the Health Care and Education Reconciliation Act of 2010 (signed into law on March 30, 2010), the Act is the product of the healthcare reform agenda of the Democratic 111th Congress and the Obama administration

Patient provider portal: A secure method of communication between the healthcare provider and the patient, just the providers, or the provider and the payer. The patient provider portal may include secure e-mail or remote access to test results, and provide patient monitoring

Patient safety: The condition of a patient being safe from harm or injury

Patient safety organization (PSO): Organizations that share the goal of improving the quality and safety of healthcare delivery; organizations eligible to become PSOs include public or private entities, profit or not-for-profit entities, provider entities such as hospital chains, and other entities that establish special components to serve as PSOs

Patient's bill of rights: The protections afforded to individuals who are undergoing medical procedures in hospitals or other healthcare facilities; *Also called* patient rights

Patient Self-Determination Act (PSDA): The federal legislation that requires healthcare facilities to provide written information on the patient's right to issue advance directives and to accept or refuse medical treatment

Patient-specific data: *See* **patent-specific/identifiable data**

Patient-specific/identifiable data: 1. Data in the health record that relate to a particular patient identified by name 2. Personal information that can be linked to a specific patient, such as age, gender, date of birth, and address-specific data

Patient's right to privacy: The justifiable expectation on the part of a patient that the information in his or her health record will be used only in the context of providing and in conjunction with healthcare services

Patient status code: A code that describes patient status at discharge or at the end of a period in form locator 17 of the CMS-1450 form

Patient summary: *See* **problem list**

Payables: Outflows of cash

Payback period: A financial method used to evaluate the value of a capital expenditure by calculating the time frame that must pass before inflow of cash from a project equals or exceeds outflow of cash

Payer of last resort (Medicaid): A Medicaid term that means Medicare pays for the services provided to individuals enrolled in both Medicare and Medicaid until Medicare benefits are exhausted and Medicaid benefits begin

Payer remittance report: A report generated by the insurance company that states the outcome of a claim and how the insurer's share of the reimbursement was determined; *See* **explanation of benefits (EOB)**

Pay for performance (P4P): 1. A type of incentive to improve clinical performance using the electronic health record that could result in additional reimbursement or eligibility for grants or other subsidies to support further HIT efforts 2. The Integrated Healthcare Association initiative in California based on the concept that physician groups would be paid for documented performance

Pay for quality (P4Q): A type of incentive to improve the quality of clinical outcomes using the electronic health record that could result in additional reimbursement or eligibility for grants or other subsidies to support further HIT efforts

Payment Error Prevention Program (PEPP): Payment compliance program established under the Sixth Scope of Work to help healthcare facilities identify simple mistakes causing payment errors; monitored by Quality Improvement Organizations (QIOs)

Payment locality: A geographic pricing area historically used by Medicare carriers to calculate physicians' customary and prevailing charges for payment of Part B services

Payment status indicator (PSI): An alphabetic code assigned to CPT/HCPCS codes to indicate whether a service or procedure is to be reimbursed under the Medicare outpatient prospective payment system

PBM: *See* **pharmacy benefits manager**

PBX: *See* **private branch exchange**

PC: *See* **professional component**

PCAOB: *See* **Public Company Accounting Oversight Board**

PCAST: *See* **President's Council of Advisors on Science and Technology**

PCDS: *See* **Patient Care Data Set**

PCG: *See* **physician care group**

PCM: *See* **primary care manager**

PCP: *See* **primary care physician** or **primary care provider**

PC Pricer: Software module in a Medicare claim-processing system, specific to certain benefits, used in pricing claims and calculating payment rates and payments, most often under prospective payment systems

PCR: *See* **physician contingency reserve**

PCU: *See* **patient care unit**

PDA: *See* **personal digital assistant**

PDCA cycle: *See* **plan-do-check-act cycle**

PDSA cycle: *See* **plan-do-study-act cycle**

PE: *See* **physician extender; practice expenses**

Pediatric patient: A patient that is at an age of minority as defined by state law at the time of discharge

Pediatric service: A service that provides diagnostic and therapeutic services for patients at age of minority

Peer review: 1. Review by like professionals, or peers, established according to an organization's medical staff bylaws, organizational policy and procedure, or the requirements of state law; the peer review system allows medical professionals to candidly critique and criticize the work of their colleagues without fear of reprisal 2. The process by which experts in the field evaluate the quality of a manuscript for publication in a scientific or professional journal

Peer-reviewed journal: A type of professional or scientific journal for which content experts evaluate articles prior to publication; *See* **refereed journal**

Peer review organization (PRO): Until 2002, a medical organization that performed a professional review of medical necessity, quality, and appropriateness of healthcare services provided to Medicare beneficiaries; now called **quality improvement organization** (QIO)

PEG: Percutaneous endoscopic gastrostomy tube

Pending: A condition during which a facility waits for payment after a bill is dropped

PEP adjustment: *See* **partial episode payment adjustment**

PEPP: *See* **Payment Error Prevention Program**

PEPPER: *See* **Program for Evaluation Payment Patterns Electronic Report**

Per case: A method of billing in which services are charged on the basis of the total service being rendered rather than by each component of the service (for example, charging for transplantation services when the organ has been procured, the transplant has been made, and aftercare has been rendered)

Percentage: A value computed on the basis of the whole divided into 100 parts

Percentage of occupancy: *See* **inpatient bed occupancy rate**

Per diem (per day): Type of prospective payment method in which the third-party payer reimburses the provider a fixed rate for each day a covered member is hospitalized

Per-diem rate: The cost per day derived by dividing total costs by the number of inpatient care days

Per-diem reimbursement: A reimbursement system based on a set payment for all of the services provided to a patient on one day rather than on the basis of actual charges

Performance counseling: Guidance provided to an individual in an attempt to improve his or her work performance

Performance evaluation: A review of an employee's job performance; *See* **performance review**

Performance improvement (PI): The continuous study and adaptation of a healthcare organization's functions and processes to increase the likelihood of achieving desired outcomes

Performance improvement council: The leadership group that oversees performance improvement activities in healthcare organizations

Performance improvement (PI) team: Members of the healthcare organization who have formed a functional or cross-functional group to examine performance issues and make recommendations for improvement

Performance indicator: A measure used by healthcare facilities to assess the quality, effectiveness, and efficiency of their services

Performance management: Encompasses all activities necessary to ensure that a company's stated goals are met in the most efficient manner

Performance measure: A quantitative tool used to assess the clinical, financial, and utilization aspects of a healthcare provider's outcomes or processes

Performance measurement: The process of comparing the outcomes of an organization, work unit, or employee against preestablished performance plans and standards

Performance measure/measurement system: System designed to improve performance by providing feedback on whether goals have been met

Performance review: An evaluation of an employee's job performance; *See* **performance evaluation**

Performance standards: The stated expectations for acceptable quality and productivity associated with a job function

Performance tests: *See* **ability (achievement) tests**

Performing: The fourth of the four steps in forming a functional team, at which point each team member is in a position to work toward achieving the team's stated goals

Perinatal death: An all-inclusive term that refers to both stillborn infants and neonatal deaths

Periodic performance review (PPR): An organizational self-assessment conducted at the halfway point between triennial on-site accreditation surveys conducted by the Joint Commission

Perioperative Nursing Dataset (PNDS): A data set developed by the Association of Perioperative Registered Nurses to identify the perioperative experience of the patient from preadmission to discharge

Peripheral: Any hardware device connected to a computer (for example, a keyboard, mouse, or printer)

Peritoneal dialysis: A continuous or intermittent procedure in which dialyzing solution is introduced into and removed from the peritoneal cavity to cleanse the body of metabolic waste products

Permanence: The quality of being in a constant, continuous state

Permanent employee: A person who is employed for an indefinite, ongoing period of time, typically long-term

Permanent national codes: HCPCS level II codes that provide a standard coding system managed by private and public insurers

Permanent variance: A financial term the refers to the difference between the budgeted amount and the actual amount of a line item that is not expected to reverse itself during a subsequent period

Per member per month (PMPM): Amount of money paid monthly for each individual enrolled in a capitation-based health insurance plan; *See* **per patient per month**

Per patient per month (PPPM): A type of managed care arrangement by which providers are paid a fixed fee in exchange for supplying all of the healthcare services an enrollee needs for a specified period of time (usually one month but sometimes one year); *See* **per member per month (PMPM)**

Personal digital assistant (PDA): A handheld microcomputer, without a hard drive, that is capable of running applications such as e-mail and providing access to data and information, such as notes, phone lists, schedules, and laboratory results, primarily through a pen device

Personal health dimension (PHD): One of three dimensions of the national health information network privacy concept that supports individuals in managing their own wellness and healthcare decision making

Personal health record (PHR): An electronic or paper health record maintained and updated by an individual for himself or herself; a tool that individuals can use to collect, track, and share past and current information about their health or the health of someone in their care

Personal/unique identifier: The unique name or numeric identifier that sets apart information for an individual person for research and administrative purposes

PERT chart: *See* **program evaluation review technique chart**

Peter Principle: A cynical belief that employees will advance to their highest level of competence, and then be promoted to their level of incompetence where they will remain (named after the 1993 book by Laurence J. Peter)

Petition for writ of certiorari: A document filed with the US Supreme Court, asking for a review of a lower court's findings

PFA: *See* **priority focus area**

PFP: *See* **priority focus process**

PFSH: *See* **Past, family, and/or social history**

PGP: *See* **pretty good privacy**

Phacoemulsification: A cataract extraction technique that uses ultrasonic waves to fragment the lens and aspirate it out of the eye

Phacofragmentation: A technique whereby the lens is broken into fragments by a mechanical means or by ultrasound

Pharmacy and therapeutics (P and T) committee: The multidisciplinary committee that oversees and monitors the drugs and therapeutics available for use, the administration of medications and therapeutics, and the positive and negative outcomes of medications and therapeutics used in a healthcare organization

Pharmacy benefits manager (PBM): The vendor selected by the Bureau of Workers' Compensation to process outpatient medication bills submitted electronically

Pharmacy information system: System that assists care providers in ordering, allocating, and administering medication; focuses on patient safety issues, especially medication errors and providing optimal patient care

PHD: *See* **personal health dimension**

PHI: *See* **protected health information**

PHII: *See* **Public Health Informatics Institute**

PHO: *See* **physician–hospital organization**

Photochemotherapy: The combination of light and chemical therapy in treating skin diseases

PHR: *See* **personal health record**

Physical access controls: 1. Security mechanisms designed to protect an organization's equipment, media, and facilities from physical damage or intrusion 2. Security mechanisms designed to prevent unauthorized physical access to health records and health record storage areas

Physical data model: The lowest level of data model with the lowest level of abstraction

Physical data repository: A repository organized into data fields, data records, and data files, storing structured, discrete, clinical, administrative, and financial data as well as unstructured, patient free-text, bitmapped, real audio, streaming video, or vector graphic data

Physical examination report: Documentation of a physician's assessment of a patient's body systems

Physical restraint: Any manual or mechanical device, material, or equipment attached or adjacent to a resident's body that restricts freedom of movement and prevents the resident's normal access to his or her own body

Physical safeguards: Measures such as locking doors to safeguard data and various media from unauthorized access and exposures; a set of four standards defined by the HIPAA Security Rule, including facility access controls, workstation use, workstation security, and device and media controls

Physical status modifier: The two-digit code (P1–P6) attached to a CPT code to describe the patient's condition and therefore the complexity of the anesthesia service

Physical therapy (PT): The field of study that focuses on physical functioning of the resident on a physician-prescribed basis

Physician assistant (PA): A healthcare professional licensed to practice medicine with physician supervision

Physician care group (PCG): Type of outpatient prospective payment method for physician services in which patients are classified into similar, homogenous categories

Physician champion: An individual who assists in communicating and educating medical staff in areas such as documentation procedures for accurate billing and appropriate EHR processes

Physician contingency reserve: *See* **withhold**

Physician extender (PE): A professional such as a physician assistant or nurse practitioner who "extends" the services of the physician to ensure continuity of care if issues or concerns arise in the long-term care setting and the physician cannot be present

Physician–hospital organization (PHO): An integrated delivery system formed by hospitals and physicians (usually through managed care contracts) that allows for cooperative activity but permits participants to retain some level of independence

Physician index: A list of patients and their physicians usually arranged according to the physician code numbers assigned by the healthcare facility

Physician–patient privilege: The legal protection from confidential communications between physicians and patients related to diagnosis and treatment being disclosed during civil and some misdemeanor litigation

Physician–patient relationship: A relationship in which the physician trusts the patient to be forthcoming and honest in providing the information necessary for diagnosis and treatment, and the patient trusts the physician to use that information responsibly, in his or her best interest, and protect it from becoming public knowledge

Physician payment reform (PPR): A legislative change in the way Medicare pays for physician services required by the Omnibus Budget Reconciliation Act of 1989, which includes a national fee schedule based on a resource-based relative value scale with geographic adjustments for differences in cost of practice, volume performance standards, and beneficiary protections

Physician profiling: A type of quality improvement and utilization management software that enables provider and payer organizations to monitor how and with what resources physicians are treating patients

Physician quality reporting system (PQRS): An incentive payment system for eligible professionals who satisfactorily report data on quality measures for covered professional services furnished to Medicare beneficiaries;

formerly known as the Physician Quality Reporting Initiative (PQRI)

Physician query process: The process by which questions are posed to a provider to obtain additional, clarifying documentation to improve the specificity and completeness of the data used to assign diagnosis and procedure codes in the patient's health record

Physician query process policy: A policy that addresses requests from physicians for additional information as part of the coding and reimbursement process

Physician's certification: A statement from a physician confirming a Medicare-eligible resident's need for long-term care services

Physician's orders: A physician's written or verbal instructions to the other caregivers involved in a patient's care

Physician work (WORK): Component or element of the relative value unit (RVU) that should cover the physician's salary. This work is the time the physician spends providing a service and the intensity with which that time is spent. The four elements of intensity are mental effort and judgment, technical skill, physical effort, and psychological stress

Physiological signal processing systems: Systems that store vector graphic data based on the human body's signals and create output based on the lines plotted between the signals' points

Physiologic effects: Cellular, tissue, or organ processes or functions altered by drugs

PI: *See* **performance improvement**

PICC: Peripherally inserted central venous catheter

Pick list: A list of options that appear below an item when clicked which a user selects to complete the computer entry; *See also* **drop-down menu**

Pictogram: A graphic technique in which pictures are used in the display of data

Picture archiving and communication system (PACS): An integrated computer system that obtains, stores, retrieves, and displays digital images (in healthcare, radiological images)

PICU: Pediatric intensive care unit

Piece-rate incentive: An adjustment of the compensation paid to a worker based on exceeding a certain level of output

Pie chart: A graphic technique in which the proportions of a category are displayed as portions of a circle (like pieces of a pie); used to show the relationship of individual parts to the whole

Pie graph: *See* **pie chart**

Pilot study: A trial run on a smaller scale; *Also called* **feasibility study**

PIN: Provider identification number

PITAC: *See* **President's Information Technology Advisory Committee**

Pixel: An abbreviation for the term *picture element*, which is defined by many tiny bits of data or points

PKI: *See* **public key infrastructure**

Placebo: A medical intervention or medication with no active ingredients

Place of service: A two-digit code used in box 24b of the CMS-1500 claim form to describe the location where the service was performed

Plain text: A message that is not encrypted; a form of text that does not support text formatting such as bold, italic, or underline; most efficient way to store text

Plaintiff: The group or person who initiates a civil lawsuit

Plan-do-check-act (PDCA) cycle: A performance improvement model developed by Walter Shewhart, but popularized in Japan by W. Edwards Deming

Plan-do-study-act (PDSA) cycle: A performance improvement model designed specifically for healthcare organizations

Planned redundancy: A disaster recovery strategy in which information technology operations are duplicated at other locations

Planning: An examination of the future and preparation of action plans to attain goals; one of the four traditional management functions

Planning stage: In performance management, the stage during which specific goals and performance standards are defined

Plan of care (POC): A term referring to Medicare home health services for homebound beneficiaries that must be delivered under a plan established by a physician

Platform: The combination of the hardware and operating system on which an application program can run

Plug-and-play: An adapter card hardware that sets connections through software rather than hardware, making hardware easier to install; a computer system's ability to detect and operate a new device as soon as it is added (for example, wireless mouse)

PMD: Primary medical doctor

PMPM: *See* **per member per month**

PMR: *See* **proportionate mortality ratio**

PNDS: *See* **perioperative nursing dataset**

P/O: *See* **prosthetics and orthotics**

POC: *See* **plan of care** or **point of care**

Point method: A method of job evaluation that places weight (points) on each of the compensable factors in a job whereby the total points associated with a job establish its relative worth and jobs that fall within a specific range of points fall into a pay grade with an associated wage

Point of care (POC): The place or location where the physician administers services to the patient

Point-of-care charting: A system whereby information is entered into the health record at the time and location of service

Point-of-care documentation: A system whereby information is entered into the health record at the time and location of service

Point-of-care information system: A computer system that captures data at the location (for example, bedside, exam room, or home) where the healthcare service is performed

Point-of-care review: *See* **open-record review**

Point-of-service (POS) healthcare insurance plan: A type of managed care plan in which enrollees are encouraged to select healthcare providers from a network of providers under contract with the plan but are also allowed to select providers outside the network and pay a larger share of the cost; *See* **open-ended HMOs**

Policies: 1. Governing principles that describe how a department or an organization is supposed to handle a specific situation or execute a specific process 2. Binding contracts issued by a healthcare insurance company to an individual or group in which the company promises to pay for healthcare to treat illness or injury; such contracts may also be referred to as **health plan agreements** and **evidence of coverage**

Policyholder: An individual or entity that purchases healthcare insurance coverage; *See* **certificate holder**; **insured**; **member**; **subscriber**

Polymorphic virus: A type of computer virus that can change its form after infecting a file

POMR: Problem-oriented medical record

Population (as related to research): The universe of data under investigation from which a sample is taken

Population-based registry: A type of registry that includes information from more than one facility in a specific geopolitical area, such as a state or region

Population-based statistics: Statistics based on a defined population rather than on a sample drawn from the same population

Population health: The capture and reporting of healthcare data that are used for public health purposes. It allows the healthcare provider to report infectious diseases, immunizations, cancer, and other reportable conditions to public health officials

Population health dimension (PHD): One of three dimensions of the National Health Information Infrastructure privacy concept that addresses protecting and promoting the health of the community

Population variance: Average of the squared deviations from the population mean

POS: Place of service or point of service

Position power: A situation in contingency theory in which the leader is perceived as having the authority to give direction

Positive relationship: A relationship in which the effect moves in the same direction; *Also called* **direct relationship**

Positivism: A philosophy of research that assumes that there is a single truth across time and place and that researchers are able to adopt a neutral, unbiased stance and establish causation; *See* **quantitative approach**

POS plan: *See* **point-of-service (POS) healthcare insurance plan**

Post-acute care: Care provided to patients who have been released from an acute care facility to recuperate at home

Postdischarge plan of care (from long-term care facility): A care plan used to help a resident discharged from the long-term care facility to adapt to his or her new living arrangement

Postmortem examination: *See* **autopsy**

Postneonatal death: The death of a live-born infant from 28 days to the end of the first year of life (364 days, 23 hours, 59 minutes from the moment of birth)

Postneonatal mortality rate: The number of deaths of persons aged 28 days up to, but not including, one year during a given time period divided by the number of live births for the same time period

Postoperative anesthesia record: Health record documentation that contains information on any unusual events or complications that occurred during surgery as well as information on the patient's condition at the conclusion of surgery and after recovery from anesthesia

Postoperative death rate: The ratio of deaths within 10 days after surgery to the total number of operations performed during a specified period of time

Postoperative infection rate: The number of infections that occur in clean surgical cases for a given time period divided by the total number of operations within the same time period

Postpartum: Occurring after childbirth

Postterm neonate: Any neonate whose birth occurs from the beginning of the first day (295th day) of the 43rd week following onset of the last menstrual period

Potentially compensable event (PCE): An event (for example, an injury, accident, or medical error) that may result in financial liability for a healthcare organization, for example, an injury, accident, or medical error

PPACA: *See* **Patient Protection and Affordable Care Act**

PPE: *See* **property, plant, and equipment**

PPO: *See* **preferred provider organization**

PPPM: *See* **per patient per month**

PPR: *See* **periodic performance review; physician payment reform**

PPS: *See* **prospective payment system**

PQRS: *See* **physician quality reporting system**

Practice expenses (PE): Element of the relative value unit (RVU) that covers the physician's overhead costs, such as employee wages, office rent, supplies, and equipment. There are two types, facility and nonfacility

Practice guidelines: Protocols of care that guide the clinical care process; *See* **Care Map**®; **clinical practice guidelines; critical paths**

Practice management system (PMS): A type of software that automates a physician office's patient appointment scheduling, registration, billing, and payroll functions

Practice without walls (PWW): *See* **group practice without walls**

Preadmission certification: *See* **prior approval (authorization)**

Preadmission review: *See* **prior approval (authorization)**

Preadmission Screening Assessment and Annual Resident Review (PASARR): A screening process for mental illness and mental retardation that must be completed prior to a prospective resident's admission to the long-term care facility

Preadmission utilization review: A type of review conducted before a patient's admission to an acute care facility to determine whether the planned service (intensity of service) or the patient's condition (severity of illness) warrants care in an inpatient setting

Preauthorization: *See* **prior approval (authorization)**

Preauthorization (precertification) number: Control number issued when a healthcare service is approved

Precertification: *See* **prior approval (authorization)**

Precision factor: The definitive tolerable error rate to be considered in calculations of productivity standards

Predecessor: A task that affects the scheduling of a successor task in a dependency relationship

Predictive modeling: A process used to identify patterns that can be used to predict the odds of a particular outcome based on the observed data

Preemption: In law, the principle that a statute at one level supercedes or is applied over the same or similar statute at a lower level (for example, the federal HIPAA privacy provisions trump the same or similar state law except when state law is more stringent)

Pre-existing condition: Any injury, disease, or physical condition occurring prior to an arbitrary date before the insured's enrollment date of coverage or any medical advice, diagnosis, care, or treatment that was recommended or received. Healthcare coverage may be denied for a period of time for a pre-existing condition, but the Health Insurance Portability and

Accountability Act constrains the use of exclusions for pre-existing conditions and establishes requirements that exclusions for pre-existing conditions must satisfy

Preferred provider organization (PPO): A managed care arrangement based on a contractual agreement between healthcare providers (professional and/or institutional) and employers, insurance carriers, or third-party administrators to provide healthcare services to a defined population of enrollees at established fees that may or may not be a discount from usual and customary or reasonable charges

Preferred term: In SNOMED CT, the description or name assigned to a concept that is used most commonly; in the UMNDS classification system, a representation of the generic product category, which is a list of preferred concepts that name devices

Pregnancy Discrimination Act: The federal legislation that prohibits discrimination against women affected by pregnancy, childbirth, or related medical conditions by requiring that affected women be treated the same as all other employees for employment-related purposes, including benefits

Pregnancy termination: The birth of a live-born or still-born infant or the expulsion or extraction of a dead fetus or other products of conception from the mother

Premium: Amount of money that a policyholder or certificate holder must periodically pay an insurer in return for healthcare coverage

Preoperative anesthesia evaluation: An assessment performed by an anesthesiologist to collect information on a patient's medical history and current physical and emotional condition that will become the basis of the anesthesia plan for the surgery to be performed

Prepartum: Occurring prior to childbirth

Prescription management: Cost-control measure that expands the use of a formulary to include patient education; electronic screening, alert, and decision-support tools; expert and referent systems; criteria for drug utilization; point-of-service order entry; electronic prescription transmission; and patient-specific medication profiles

Present on admission (POA): A condition present at the time of inpatient admission

Present value: A value that targets the current dollar investment and interest-rate needs to achieve a particular investment goal

President's Council of Advisors on Science and Technology: An advisory group of the nation's leading scientists and engineers who directly advise the President and the Executive Office of the President; makes policy recommendations in the many areas where understanding of science, technology, and innovation is key to strengthening the economy and forming policy

President's Information Technology Advisory Committee (PITAC): A committee that advises the federal administration on information technology, including EHR interoperability issues; part of the President's Council of Advisors on Science and Technology (PCAST)

Preterm infant: An infant with a birth weight between 1,000 and 2,499 grams and/or a gestation between 28 and 37 completed weeks

Preterm neonate: Any neonate whose birth occurs through the end of the last day of the 38th week (266th day) following onset of the last menstrual period

Pretty good privacy (PGP): A type of encryption software that uses public key cryptology and digital signatures

Prevalence rate: The proportion of people in a population who have a particular disease at a specific point in time or over a specified period of time

Prevalence study: *See* **cross-sectional study**

Preventive controls: Internal controls implemented prior to an activity and designed to stop an error from happening

Primary analysis: The analysis of original research data by the researchers who collected them

Primary care: The continuous and comprehensive care provided at first contact with the healthcare provider in an ambulatory care setting

Primary care manager (PCM): The healthcare provider assigned to a TRICARE beneficiary

Primary care physician (PCP): 1. Physician who provides, supervises, and coordinates the healthcare of a member and who manages referrals to other healthcare providers and utilization of healthcare services both inside and outside a managed care plan. Family and general practitioners, internists, pediatricians, and obstetricians and gynecologists are primary care physicians

2. The physician who makes the initial diagnosis of a patient's medical condition; *See* **primary care provider**

Primary care provider (PCP): Healthcare provider who provides, supervises, and coordinates the healthcare of a member; primary care providers can be family and general practitioners, internists, pediatricians, and obstetricians and gynecologists; other PCPs are nurse practitioners and physician assistants; *See* **primary care physician**

Primary data source (in healthcare): A record developed by healthcare professionals in the process of providing patient care

Primary diagnosis: *See* **principal diagnosis**

Primary insurer (payer): The insurance company responsible for making the first payment on a claim; *See* **secondary insurer**

Primary key: An explanatory notation that uniquely identifies each row in a database table; *See* **key field**

Primary patient record: *See* **health record**

Primary record of care: *See* **health record**

Primary research: Data collected specifically for a study

Primary source: An original work of a researcher who conducted an investigation

Primary source system: An information system that is part of the overall clinical information system in which documentation is most commonly first entered or generated

Principal diagnosis: The disease or condition that was present on admission, was the principal reason for admission, and received treatment or evaluation during the hospital stay or visit *or* the reason established after study to be chiefly responsible for occasioning the admission of the patient to the hospital for care; *See* **most significant diagnosis**

Principal investigator: The individual with primary responsibility for the design and conduct of a research project

Principal procedure: The procedure performed for the definitive treatment of a condition (as opposed to a procedure performed for diagnostic or exploratory purposes) or for care of a complication

Print file: Output from a computer system that generates a file containing an image of information that can be printed

Prior approval (authorization): Process of obtaining approval from a healthcare insurance company before receiving healthcare services; *Also called* **precertification**

Priority focus area (PFA): One of 14 areas that the Joint Commission considers vital in the successful operation of a hospital; includes processes, systems, and structures that have a substantial effect on patient care services

Priority focus process (PFP): A process used by the Joint Commission to collect, analyze, and create information about a specific organization being accredited in order to customize the accreditation process

Privacy: The quality or state of being hidden from, or undisturbed by, the observation or activities of other persons, or freedom from unauthorized intrusion; in healthcare-related contexts, the right of a patient to control disclosure of protected health information

Privacy Act of 1974: A law that requires federal agencies to safeguard personally identifiable records and provides individuals with certain privacy rights

Privacy (research) board: A group formed by a HIPAA-covered entity to review research studies where authorization waivers are requested and to ensure the HIPAA privacy rights of research subjects

Privacy officer: A position mandated under the HIPAA Privacy Rule—covered entities must designate an individual to be responsible for developing and implementing privacy policies and procedures

Privacy Protection Study Commission: A commission established to review the weaknesses of the Privacy Act of 1974, evaluate the statute, and issue a report containing recommendations for its improvement to grant greater protections

Privacy Rule: The federal regulations created to implement the privacy requirements of the simplification subtitle of the Health Insurance Portability and Accountability Act of 1996; effective in 2002; afforded patients certain rights to and about their protected health information

Privacy standards: Rules, conditions, or requirements developed to ensure the privacy of patient information

Private branch exchange (PBX): A switching system for telephones on private extension lines that allows access to the public telephone network

Private key: In cryptography, an asymmetric algorithm restricted to one entity; *See* **cryptography**; **key**; **public key**

Private law: The collective rules and principles that define the rights and duties of people and private businesses

Private right of action: 1. The right of an injured person to secure redress for violation of his or her rights 2. A legal right to maintain an action growing out of a given transaction or state of facts and based thereon or a legal term pertaining to remedy and relief through judicial procedure

Private, unrestricted fee-for-service plan: A prepaid health insurance plan that allows beneficiaries to select private healthcare providers

Privilege: The professional relationship between patients and specific groups of caregivers that affects the patient's health record and its contents as evidence; the services or procedures, based on training and experience, that an individual physician is qualified to perform; a right granted to a user, program, or process that allows access to certain files or data in a system

Privileged communication: The protection afforded to the recipients of professional services that prohibits medical practitioners, lawyers, and other professionals from disclosing the confidential information that they learn in their capacity as professional service providers

Privileging process: The process of evaluating a physician's or other licensed independent practitioner's quality of medical practice and determining the services or procedures he or she is qualified to perform

PRO: *See* **peer review organization**

Probate court: A state court that handles wills and settles estates

Probationary period: A period of time in which the skills of a potential employee's work are assessed before he or she assumes full-time employment

Problem list: A list of illnesses, injuries, and other factors that affect the health of an individual patient, usually identifying the time of occurrence or identification and resolution; *See* **patient summary**; **summary list**

Problem-oriented health record format: A health record documentation approach in which the physician defines each clinical problem individually

Problem-oriented health record: Patient record in which clinical problems are defined and documented individually; *Also called* **problem-oriented medical record**

Problem-oriented medical record (POMR): *See* **problem-oriented health record**

Procedural codes: The numeric or alphanumeric characters used to classify and report the medical procedures and services performed for patients

Procedural risk: A professionally recognized risk that a given procedure may induce functional impairment, injury, morbidity, or mortality

Procedure: 1. A document that describes the steps involved in performing a specific function 2. An action of a medical professional for treatment or diagnosis of a medical condition 3. The steps taken to implement a policy; *See* **surgical procedure**

Procedures and services (outpatient): All medical procedures and services of any type (including history, physical examination, laboratory, x-ray or radiograph, and others) that are performed pertinent to the patient's reasons for the encounter, all therapeutic services performed at the time of the encounter, and all preventive services and procedures performed at the time of the encounter

Process: A systematic series of actions taken to create a product or service

Process and workflow modeling: The process of creating a representation of the actions and information required to perform a function, including decomposition diagrams, dependency diagrams, and data flow diagrams

Process improvement: A series of actions taken to identify, analyze, and improve existing processes

Process improvement team: An interdepartmental task force formed to redesign or change and improve shared processes and procedures

Process indicators: Specific measures that enable the assessment of the steps taken in rendering a service; *Also called* **process measures**

Process measures: Measures that focus on a process that leads to a certain outcome, meaning that a scientific basis exists for believing that the process, when executed well, will increase the probability of achieving a desired outcome

Process redesign: The steps in which focused data are collected and analyzed, the process is changed to incorporate the knowledge gained from the data collected, the new process is implemented, and the staff is educated about the new process

Product Code: The part of the National Drug Code that identifies a specific strength, dosage form, and formulation for a particular drug

Product trade name: Name (also referred to as catalog name) assigned or supplied by the labelers (firms) as required under the Food, Drug, and Cosmetic Act

Productivity: A unit of performance defined by management in quantitative standards

Productivity bonus: A monetary incentive used to encourage employees to improve their output

Productivity indicators: A set of measures designed to routinely monitor the output and quality of products and/or services provided by an individual, an organization, or one of its constituent parts; used to help determine status of a productivity bonus

Productivity software: A type of computer software used for word-processing, spreadsheet, and database management applications

Professional certification organizations: Private societies and membership organizations that establish professional qualification requirements and clinical practice standards for specific areas of medicine, nursing, and allied health professions

Professional component (PC): 1. The portion of a healthcare procedure performed by a physician 2. A term generally used in reference to the elements of radiological procedures performed by a physician

Professional standards review organization (PSRO): An organization responsible for determining whether the care and services provided to hospital inpatients were medically necessary and met professional standards in the context of eligibility for reimbursement under the Medicare and Medicaid programs

Profiling: 1. A measurement of the quality, utilization, and cost of medical resources provided by physicians that is made by employers, third-party payers, government entities, and other purchasers of healthcare 2. A technique used to compare the activities of one or more healthcare providers

Profit: The difference between revenues and expenses used to build reserves for contingencies and long-term capital improvements; *See* **net income**

Profitability index: An index used to prioritize investment opportunities, where the present value of the cash inflows is divided by the present value of the cash outflows for each investment and the results are compared

Profit and loss statement: *See* **statement of revenue and expenses**

Pro forma: An estimate

Prognosis: The probable outcome of an illness, including the likelihood of improvement or deterioration in the severity of the illness, the likelihood for recurrence, and the patient's probable life expectancy

Program budget: *See* **milestone budget**

Program evaluation and review technique (PERT) chart: A project management tool that diagrams a project's time lines and tasks as well as their interdependencies

Program for Evaluation Payment Patterns Electronic Report (PEPPER): A benchmarking database maintained by the Texas Medical Foundation that supplies individual QIOs with hospital data to determine state benchmarks and monitor hospital compliance

Program officer: The person who leads a specific request for applications (RFA) or request for proposals (RFP) and addresses any questions the investigators may have while developing a proposal

Programmed decision: An automated decision made by people or computers based on a situation being so stable and recurrent that decision rules can be applied to it

Programmers: Individuals primarily responsible for writing program codes and developing applications, typically performing the function of systems development and working closely with system analysts

Programming language: A set of words and symbols that allows programmers to tell the computer what operations to follow

Programs of All-Inclusive Care for the Elderly (PACE): A state option legislated by the Balanced Budget Act of 1997 that provides an alternative to institutional care for individuals 55 years old or older who require the level of care provided by nursing facilities

Progress notes: The documentation of a patient's care, treatment, and therapeutic response, which is entered into the health record by each of the clinical professionals involved in a patient's care, including nurses, physicians, therapists, and social workers

Progressive discipline: A four-step process for shaping employee behavior to conform to the requirements of the employee's job position that begins with a verbal caution and progresses to written reprimand, suspension, and dismissal upon subsequent offenses

Prohibited abbreviations: Acronyms, abbreviations, and symbols that cannot be used in health records because they are prone to misinterpretation

Project charter: *See* **statement of work**

Project components: Related parameters of scope, resources, and scheduling with regard to a project

Project definition: First step in the project management life cycle that sets expectations for the what, when, and how of a project the organization wants to undertake

Project deliverables: The tangible end results of a project

Project management: A formal set of principles and procedures that help control the activities associated with implementing a usually large undertaking to achieve a specific goal, such as an information system project

Project management life cycle: The period in which the processes involved in carrying out a project are completed, including project definition, project planning and organization, project tracking and analysis, project revisions, change control, and communication

Project management software: A type of application software that provides the tools to track a project

Project network: The relationship between tasks in a project that determines the overall finish date

Project office: A support function for project management best practices

Project plan: A plan consisting of a list of the tasks to be performed in a project, a defined order in which they will occur, task start and finish dates, and the resource effort needed to complete each task

Project schedule: The portion of the project plan that deals specifically with task start and finish dates

Project scope: 1. The intention of a project 2. The range of a project's activities or influence

Project team: A collection of individuals assigned to work on a project

Promotion: The act of being raised in position or rank

Property, plant, and equipment (PPE): *See* **capital assets**

Proportion: The relation of one part to another or to the whole with respect to magnitude, quantity, or degree

Proportionate mortality ratio (PMR): The total number of deaths due to a specific cause during a given time period divided by the total number of deaths due to all causes

Prosecutor: An attorney who prosecutes a defendant accused of a crime on behalf of a local, state, or federal government

Prospective payment: A method of determining reimbursement based on predetermined factors, not individual services

Prospective payment method: Type of episode-of-care reimbursement in which the third-party payer establishes the payment rates for healthcare services in advance for a specific time period

Prospective payment system (PPS): A type of reimbursement system that is based on preset payment levels rather than actual charges billed after the service has been provided; specifically, one of several Medicare reimbursement systems based on predetermined payment rates or periods and linked to the anticipated intensity of services delivered as well as the beneficiary's condition; *See* **acute care prospective payment system; home health prospective payment system; outpatient prospective payment system; skilled nursing facility prospective payment system**

Prospective reimbursement: *See* **prospective payment system**

Prospective study: A study designed to observe outcomes or events that occur after the identification of a group of subjects to be studied

Prospective utilization review: A review of a patient's health records before admission to determine the necessity of admission to an acute care facility and to determine or satisfy benefit coverage requirements

Prosthetics and orthotics (P/O): A collective term that refers to the artificial extremities, augmentation devices, and mechanical appliances used in orthopedic care

Protected health information (PHI): Individually identifiable health information, transmitted electronically or maintained in any other form, that is created or received by a healthcare provider or any other entity subject to HIPAA requirements

Protective order: Any court order or decree whose purpose is to protect a person from personal harassment or service of process or discovery

Protocol: In healthcare, a detailed plan of care for a specific medical condition based on investigative studies; in medical research, a rule or procedure to be followed in a clinical trial; in a computer network, a rule or procedure used to address and ensure delivery of data

Provider: Physician, clinic, hospital, nursing home, or other healthcare entity (second party) that delivers healthcare services

Provider-based entity: A provider of healthcare services, a rural health clinic, or a federally qualified health clinic, as defined in section 405-2401 of the *Code of Federal Regulations*, that is either created or acquired by a main provider for the purpose of furnishing healthcare services under the name, ownership, and administrative and financial control of the main provider, in accordance with the provisions of the proposed rule

Provider-based status: The relationship between a main provider and a provider-based entity or a department of a provider that complies with the provisions of the final rule on ambulatory payment classifications

Provider network organization: An organization that performs prospective, concurrent, and retrospective reviews of healthcare services provided to its enrollees

Provider-sponsored organization (PSO): Type of point-of-service plan in which the physicians that practice in a regional or community hospital organize the plan

PSDA: *See* **Patient Self-Determination Act**

PSI: *See* **payment status indicator**

PSO: *See* **patient safety organization**; **provider-sponsored organization**

PSRO: *See* **professional standards review organization**

Psychiatric hospital: A hospital that provides diagnostic and treatment services to patients with mental or behavioral disorders

Psychiatry: The study, treatment, and prevention of mental disorders

Psychotherapy notes: Notes recorded in any medium by a mental health professional to document or analyze the contents of conversations between therapists and clients during private or group counseling sessions

PT: *See* **physical therapy**

PTCA: Percutaneous transluminal coronary angioplasty

P/T committee: *See* **pharmacy and therapeutics committee**

Public assistance: A monetary subsidy provided to financially needy individuals; *Also called* welfare

Public Company Accounting Oversight Board (PCAOB): A not-for-profit organization that oversees the work of auditors of public companies

Public health: An area of healthcare that deals with the health of populations in geopolitical areas, such as states and counties

Public Health Informatics Institute (PHII): A cooperative of public health services, health information systems, and informatics experts established to develop health information systems for public and population health purposes

Public health services (PHS): Services concerned primarily with the health of entire communities and population groups

Public key: In cryptography, an asymmetric algorithm made publicly available to unlock a coded message; *See* **cryptography**; **key**; **private key**

Public key infrastructure (PKI): A system of digital certificates and other registration authorities that verify and authenticate the validity of each party involved in a secure transaction

Public law: A type of legislation that involves the government and its relations with individuals and business organizations

Public Law 104-191: The alternate name for the Health Insurance Portability and Accountability Act (HIPAA) passed in 1996; *See* **Health Insurance Portability and Accountability Act of 1996**

Puerperal: The period immediately following childbirth

Pull-down menu: The design of a data-entry screen of a computer in which categories of functions or structured data elements may be accessed through that category element in a list format

Pull list: A list of requests for records to be pulled for review during the audit process

Purchase order: A paper document or electronic screen on which all details of an intended purchase are reported, including authorizations

Purged records: Patient health records that have been removed from the active file area

Purposive sampling: A strategy of qualitative research in which researchers use their expertise to select representative units and unrepresentative units to capture a wide array of perspectives

Push technology: A type of active computer technology that sends information directly to the end user as the information becomes available

PWW: *See* **group practice without walls**

Q

QA: *See* **quality assurance**
QDWIs: *See* **qualified disabled and working individuals**
QI: *See* **quality improvement**
QIO: *See* **quality improvement organization**
QIs: *See* **qualifying individuals**
QI toolbox techniques: Tools that facilitate the collection, display, and analysis of data and information and that help team members stay focused, including cause-and-effect diagrams, graphic presentations, and others

QMBs: *See* **qualified Medicare beneficiaries**
Qualified disabled and working individuals (QDWIs): Medicare beneficiaries who are eligible for assistance, including disabled and working people who previously qualified for Medicare because of disability but lost entitlement because of their return to work despite the disability

Qualified electronic health record: An EHR on an individual that includes patient demographic and clinical health information and has the capacity to provide clinical decision support; to support physician order entry; to capture and query information relevant to healthcare quality; and to exchange electronic health information with, and integrate such information from, other sources

Qualified Medicare beneficiaries (QMBs): Medicare beneficiaries who have resources at or below twice the standard allowed under the Social Security Income program and incomes at or below 100 percent of the federal poverty level

Qualifying circumstances: Unusual situations such as extreme age, total body hypothermia, controlled hypotension, and emergency situations that complicate the provision of anesthesia

Qualifying individuals (QIs): Medicare beneficiaries whose incomes are at least 120 percent, but less than 175 percent, of the federal poverty level

Qualitative analysis: A review of the health record to ensure that standards are met and to determine the adequacy of entries documenting the quality of care

Qualitative approach: *See* **naturalism**

Qualitative research: A philosophy of research that assumes that multiple contextual truths exist and bias is always present; *Also called* **naturalism**

Qualitative standards: Service standards in the context of setting expectations for how well or how soon work or a service will be performed

Quality: The degree or grade of excellence of goods or services, including, in healthcare, meeting expectations for outcomes of care

Quality assurance (QA): A set of activities designed to measure the quality of a service, product, or process with remedial action, as needed, to maintain a desired standard

Quality gap: The difference between approved standards, criteria, or expectations in any type of process and actual results

Quality improvement (QI): A set of activities that measures the quality of a service or product through systems or process evaluation and then implements revised processes that result in better healthcare outcomes for patients, based on standards of care

Quality improvement organization (QIO): An organization that performs medical peer review of Medicare and Medicaid claims, including review of validity of hospital diagnosis and procedure coding information; completeness, adequacy, and quality of care; and appropriateness of prospective payments for outlier cases and nonemergent use of the emergency room. Until 2002, called peer review organization

Quality improvement process: An approach undertaken to improve healthcare delivery that involves two principal steps: problem identification and process redesign

Quality indicator (QI): A standard against which actual care may be measured to identify a level of performance for that standard

Quality management: Evaluation of the quality of healthcare services and delivery using standards and guidelines developed by various entities, including the government and independent accreditation organizations

Quality measures: *See* **performance measure**

Quality review organization: A quality improvement organization or an accreditation organization

Quantitative analysis: A review of the health record to determine its completeness and accuracy

Quantitative approach: A philosophy of research that assumes that there is a single truth across time and place and that researchers are able to adopt a neutral, unbiased stance and establish causation; *See* **positivism**

Quantitative audit: An audit that compares a report of services billed for a specific client and within a specific time frame against the health record documentation; *Also called* **billing audit**

Quantitative research: *See* **quantitative approach**

Quartile: The fourth equal part of a distribution

Quasi experimental design: *See* **causal-comparative research**

Questionable covered procedure: A procedure that may or may not be covered, depending on the patient's diagnosis and other factors

Questionnaire: A type of survey in which the members of the population are questioned through the use of electronic or paper forms

Queuing theory: An operations management technique for examining customer flow and designing ideal wait or scheduling times

Quintile: Portion of a frequency distribution containing one-fifth of the total cases

Qui tam: The "whistleblower" provisions of the False Claims Act which provides that private persons, known as relators, may enforce the Act by filing a complaint, under seal, alleging fraud committed against the government

Quota sampling: A sampling technique where the population is first segmented into mutually exclusive subgroups, just as in stratified sampling, and then judgment is used to select the subjects or units from each segment based on a specified proportion

Quotient: The number resulting from the division of one number by another

RA: *See* **remittance advice**

RAC: *See* **recovery audit contractor**

Radioactive ribbon: A small plastic tube (ribbon) that has radioactive sources spaced at regular lengths along it. Ribbon refers to temporary interstitial placement

Radioactive source: Radioactive elements packaged in a small configuration used for permanent implantation into tumors

Radio frequency identification (RFID): An automatic recognition technology that uses a device attached to an object to transmit data to a receiver and does not require direct contact

Radioimmunoassay: A procedure that combines the use of radioactive chemicals and antibodies to detect hormones and drugs in a patient's blood

Radioimmunoprecipitation assay (RIPA): A confirmatory blood test that is used to detect HIV infection. It is used when HIV antibody levels are very low or difficult to detect

Radiology information system (RIS): A system that collects, stores, and provides information on radiological tests such as ultrasound, magnetic resonance imaging, and positron emission tomography. The RIS also supports other radiological procedures performed in radiology such as ultrasound-guided biopsies and upper gastrointestinal series

R-ADT: *See* **Registration data of the admission, discharge, transfer**

RAI: *See* **resident assessment instrument**

RAID: *See* **redundant array of inexpensive disks**

Randomization: The assignment of subjects to experimental or control groups based on chance

Randomized clinical trial (RCT): A special type of clinical trial in which the researchers follow strict rules to randomly assign patients to groups

Random sampling: An unbiased selection of subjects that includes methods such as simple random sampling, stratified random sampling, systematic sampling, and cluster sampling

Range: A measure of variability between the smallest and largest observations in a frequency distribution

Ranked data: A type of ordinal data where the group of observations is first arranged from highest to lowest according to magnitude and then assigned numbers that correspond to each observation's place in the sequence

RAP: *See* **request for anticipated payment; resident assessment protocol**

Raster image: A digital image or digital data made up of pixels in a horizontal and vertical grid or a matrix instead of lines plotted between a series of points

Rate: A measure used to compare an event over time; a comparison of the number of times an event did happen (numerator) with the number of times an event could have happened (denominator)

Rate of return method: A method used to justify a proposed capital expenditure in which the organization tries to find out what rate of return it would get if it invests in a particular project

Rating stage: In performance management, the fourth of five steps during which specific performance criteria are evaluated

Ratio: 1. A calculation found by dividing one quantity by another 2. A general term that can include a number of specific measures such as proportion, percentage, and rate

Ratio analysis: Mathematical computations that compare elements of an organization's financial statements to past and future performance trends and industry benchmarks

Ratio data: Data that may be displayed by units of equal size and placed on a scale starting with zero and thus can be manipulated mathematically (for example, 0, 5, 10, 15, 20)

Ratio-level data: Data with a defined unit of measure, a real zero point, and with equal intervals between successive values; *Also called* **ratio data;** *See* **interval-level data**

Ratio scale: Continuous data having both equal intervals and an absolute zero point

RAVEN: *See* **Resident Assessment Validation and Entry**

RBAC: *See* **role-based access control**

RBRVS: *See* **resource-based relative value scale**

R&C: *See* **reasonable and customary charges**

RCT: *See* **randomized clinical trial**

RDBMS: *See* **relational database management system**

Read Codes: The former name of the United Kingdom's CTV-3 codes; named for James Read, the physician who originally devised the system to organize computer-based patient data in his primary care practice. *See* **Clinical Terms Version 3 (CTV3)**

Readiness assessment: An evaluation of a healthcare organization's infrastructure to identify and capture information on what must be addressed and where to apply resources in preparation for change such as an EHR implementation or ICD-10 transition

Reagent: Any substance added to a solution of another substance to participate in a chemical reaction

Real audio data: The storing, manipulating, and displaying of sound in a computer-readable format; *Also called* **sound data**

Reasonable and customary charges (R&C): The amounts charged by healthcare providers consistent with charges from similar providers for identical or similar services in a given locale; *See* **usual, customary, and reasonable**

Reasonable care: The degree of care that a reasonably prudent person would exercise in the same or similar circumstances

Reasons for encounter (RFE): In the international classification of primary care (ICPC) system, the subjective experience by the patient of the problem or the "reason for encounter"

Reattachment: Putting back in or on all or a portion of a separated body part to its normal location or other suitable location. During this procedure the vascular circulation and nervous pathways may or may not be reestablished

Rebasing: The redetermination of the ambulatory payment classification weights to reflect changes in relative resource consumption

Rebill: The act of resubmitting a corrected bill to the payer after it has been rejected

Recalibration: The adjustment of all ambulatory payment classification weights to reflect changes in relative resource consumption

Recap: Abbreviation of *recapitulation*

Recapitulation: A concise summary of data

Receivables: Amounts of money coming into the organization; *Also called* **assets**

Record completion: The process whereby healthcare professionals are able to access, complete, and/or authenticate a specific patient's medical information

Record custodian: The person who has been designated responsible for the care, custody, and control of the health record for such persons or institutions that prepare and maintain records of healthcare. They are authorized to certify records and supervise all inspections, releases, or duplication of records. The custodian may be called to testify to the admissibility of the record, verify timeliness, and verify that normal business practices were used to develop and maintain the health record

Record locator service (RLS): A service that indicates where a given patient may have health information, using probability equations

Record of Care, Treatment, and Services: A chapter in the Joint Commission accreditation manual that provides standards for managing health information specifically addressing the clinical record itself

Record processing: The processes that encompass the creation, maintenance, and updating of each patient's medical record

Record reconciliation: The process of assuring that all the records of discharged patients have been received by the HIM department for processing

Records disaster recovery policy: A policy that establishes how records should be handled in a disaster such as fire or flood

Records purging policy: A policy that is used in conjunction with the off-site storage policy and retention policy

Records retention policy: A policy that specifies the length of time that health records are kept as required by law and operational needs

Recovery Act: *See* **American Recovery and Reinvestment Act of 2009**

Recovery audit contractor (RAC): A governmental program whose goal is to identify improper payments made on claims of healthcare services provided to Medicare beneficiaries. Improper payments may be overpayments or underpayments

Recovery room record: A type of health record documentation used by nurses to document the patient's reaction to anesthesia and condition after surgery; *Also called* recovery room report

Recruitment: The process of finding, soliciting, and attracting employees

Recurrence: A return of symptoms as part of the natural progress of a disease

Red Flag Rules: A set of FTC regulations that require certain entities to develop and implement identity theft prevention programs

Red flags: Suspicious documents, information, or behaviors that indicate the possibility of identity theft

Redisclosure: The release, transfer, provision of access to, or divulging in any other manner of patient health information that was generated by an external source to others outside of the organization and its workforce members

Redundancy: As data is entered and processed by one server, data is simultaneously being entered and processed by a second server. The concept of building a backup computer system that is an exact version of the primary system and that can replace it in the event of a primary system failure

Redundant arrays of independent (or inexpensive) disks (RAID): A method of ensuring data security

Reengineering: Fundamental rethinking and radical redesign of business processes to achieve significant performance improvements

Refereed journal: *See* **peer-reviewed journal**

Reference check: Contact made with an individual that a prospective employee has listed to provide a favorable account of his or her work performance or personal attributes

Reference data: Information that interacts with the care of the individual or with the healthcare delivery system, such as a formulary, protocol, care plan, clinical alert, or reminder

Reference terminology: A set of concepts and relationships that provide a common consultation point for the comparison and aggregation of data about the entire healthcare process, recorded by multiple individuals, systems, or institutions

Referral: A request by a provider for a patient under the provider's care to be evaluated and/or treated by another provider

Referred outpatient: An outpatient who is provided special diagnostic or therapeutic services by a hospital on an ambulatory basis but whose medical care remains the responsibility of the referring physician

Refined case-based payment method: Case-based payment method enhanced to include patients from all age groups or from regions of the world with varying mixes of diseases and differing patterns of healthcare delivery

Reflective learning cycle: Uses awareness to formulate an interpretation of what has been observed, considers what difference can be made by applying what has been learned, and executes the efforts toward change through deliberate action. A cycle of reflection, interpretation, application of learning, and action that is the basis of total quality management and other continuous improvement philosophies

Refreezing: Lewin's last stage of change in which the new behaviors are reinforced to become as stable and institutionalized as the previous status quo behaviors

Regenstrief LOINC Mapping Assistant (RELMA): A free Microsoft Windows software download that provides LOINC users help in working with LOINC database files

Regenstrief Medical Records System (RMRS): One of the nation's first electronic medical record systems and the keystone of Regenstrief Institute activities

Regional health information network (RHIN): System that links various healthcare information systems in a region together so that patients, healthcare institutions, and other entities can share clinical information

Regional health information organization (RHIO): A health information organization that brings together healthcare stakeholders within a defined geographic area and governs health information exchange among them for the purpose of improving health and care in the community

Regional home health intermediaries (RHHI): Private companies that contract with Medicare to pay home health bills and check on the quality of home healthcare

Registered health information administrator (RHIA): A type of certification granted after completion of an AHIMA-accredited four-year program in health information management and a credentialing examination

Registered health information technician (RHIT): A type of certification granted after completion of an AHIMA-accredited two-year program in health information management and a credentialing examination

Registered nurse (RN): A graduate nurse who has passed a national licensing examination

Registration: The act of enrolling

Registration data of the admission, discharge, transfer (R-ADT): A type of administrative information system that stores demographic information and performs functionality related to registration, admission, discharge, and transfer of patients within the organization

Registry: A collection of care information related to a specific disease, condition, or procedure that makes health record information available for analysis and comparison

Regression analysis: Statistical technique that uses an independent variable to predict the value of a dependent variable. In the inpatient psychiatric facility prospective payment system (IPF PPS), patient demographics and length of stay (independent variables) were used to predict cost of care (dependent variable)

Regulation: A rule established by an administrative agency of government. The difference between a statute and a regulation is regulations must be followed by any healthcare organization participating in the related program. Administrative agencies are responsible for implementing and managing the programs instituted by state and federal statutes

Rehabilitation: The process of restoring the disabled insured to maximum physical, mental, and vocational independence and productivity (commensurate with their limitations) through the identification and development of residual capabilities, job modifications, or retraining; *Also called* rehabilitation care

Rehabilitation Act: Federal legislation passed in 1973 to protect handicapped employees against discrimination

Rehabilitation facility: Facility specializing in the restorative processes and therapies that develop and maintain self-sufficient functioning consistent with individuals' capabilities. Rehabilitative services restore function after an illness or injury. Services are provided by psychiatrists, nurses, and physical, occupational, and speech therapists

Rehabilitation impairment category (RIC): Clusters of impairment group codes (IGCs) that represent similar impairments and diagnoses. RICs are the larger umbrella division within the inpatient rehabilitation facility prospective payment system (IRF PPS). From the RICs, the case-mix groups (CMGs) are determined

Rehabilitation services: Health services provided to assist patients in achieving and maintaining their optimal level of function, self-care, and independence after some type of disability

Reimbursement: Compensation or repayment for healthcare services

Reinforcement: The process of increasing the probability of a desired response through reward

Rejection: The process of having a submitted bill not accepted by the payer, although corrections can be made and the claim resubmitted

Relational database: A type of database that stores data in predefined tables made up of rows and columns

Relational database management system (RDBMS): A database management system in which data are organized and managed as a collection of tables

Relational online analytical processing (ROLAP): A data access methodology that provides users with various drill-down and business analysis capabilities similar to online analytical processing

Relationship: A type of connection between two terms

Relative frequency: The percentage of times that a character appears in a data set

Relative risk (RR): A ratio that compares the risk of disease between two groups; *Also called* risk ratio

Relative value scale (RVS): System designed to permit comparisons of the resources needed or appropriate prices for various units of service, taking into account labor, skill, supplies, equipment, space, and other costs for each procedure or service; specifically refers to relative physician work values developed by the Harvard University relative value scale study

Relative value study (RVS): A guide that shows the relationship among the time, resources, competency, experience, severity, and other factors necessary to perform procedures

Relative value unit (RVU): A number assigned to a procedure that describes its difficulty and expense in relationship to other procedures by assigning weights to such factors as personnel, time, and level of skill; *See* **geographic practice cost index; malpractice; physician work; practice expenses; resource-based relative value scale**

Relative weight (RW): Assigned weight that reflects the relative resource consumption associated with a payment classification or group; higher payments are associated with higher relative weights

Release: Freeing a body part from an abnormal physical constraint by cutting or by use of force. Coded to the body part being freed in ICD-10-PCS

Release and disclosure: The processes that make health record information available to legitimate users

Release of information (ROI): The process of disclosing patient-identifiable information from the health record to another party

Relevance: How applicable information is to some matter

Reliability: A measure of consistency of data items based on their reproducibility and an estimation of their error of measurement

RELMA: *See* **Regenstrief LOINC Mapping Assistant**

Reminder: A prompt based on a set of rules that displays on the computer workstation, similar to a recommendation

Remittance advice (RA): An explanation of payments (for example, claim denials) made by third-party payers

Remote patient monitoring device: A device that enables a healthcare provider to monitor and treat a patient from a remote location

Removal: Taking out or off a device from a body part in ICD-10-PCS

Repair: Restoring, to the extent possible, a body part to its normal anatomical structure and function. It also functions as the "not elsewhere classified (NEC)" root operation and is to be used when the procedure performed does not meet the definition of one of the other root operations in ICD-10-PCS

Replacement: Putting in or on biological or synthetic material that physically takes the place and/or function of all or a portion of a body part in ICD-10-PCS

Reportable adverse event: An unintended act, either of omission or commission, or an act that does not achieve its intended outcome

Report cards: A method used by managed care organizations (and other healthcare sectors) to report cost and quality of care provided

Report generation: The process of analyzing, organizing, and presenting recorded patient information for authentication and inclusion in the patient's healthcare record; the formatting and/or structuring of captured information

Reposition: Moving all or a portion of a body part to its normal location or other suitable location in ICD-10-PCS

Repository: A data structure where data are stored for subsequent use by multiple, disparate systems

Repudiation: A situation in which a user or system denies having performed some action, such as modifying information

Request for anticipated payment (RAP): The first of two Centers for Medicare and Medicaid Services forms used at the opening of a prospective payment system episode to ask for one of two split-percentage payments; not a claim according to Medicare statutes

Request for applications (RFA): The project announcement that describes the project and encourages researchers to apply; it may list additional criteria specific to the announcement; *See* **request for proposal**

Request for information (RFI): A written communication often sent to a comprehensive list of vendors during the design phase of the systems development life cycle to ask for general product information

Request for production: A discovery device used to compel another party to produce documents and other items or evidence important to a lawsuit

Request for proposal (RFP): A type of business correspondence asking for very specific product and contract information that is often sent to a narrow list of vendors that have been preselected after a review of requests for information during the design phase of the systems development life cycle; *See* **request for applications**

Request restrictions: Under the Privacy Rule, the right of an individual to request that a covered entity limit the uses and disclosures of PHI to carry out treatment, payment, or healthcare operations

Required standards: The implementation specifications of the HIPAA Security Rule that are designated "required" rather than "addressable;" required standards must be present for the covered entity to be in compliance

Requisition: A request from an authorized health record user to gain access to a medical record

Research: An inquiry process aimed at discovering new information about a subject or revising old information. Investigation or experimentation aimed at the discovery and interpretation of facts, revision of accepted theories or laws in the light of new facts, or practical application of such new or revised theories or laws; the collecting of information about a particular subject

Research data: Data used for the purpose of answering a proposed question or testing a hypothesis

Research method: The particular strategy used by a researcher to collect, analyze, and present data

Research methodology: A set of procedures or strategies used by researchers to collect, analyze, and present data

Resection: Cutting out or off, without replacement, all of a body part. Includes all of a body part or any subdivision of a body part that has its own body part value in ICD-10-PCS

Reserves: Unused profits from a not-for-profit organization that stay in the business

Residence: A patient's full address and zip code

Residency program: An accredited program whereby a hospital sponsors graduate medical education for physicians in training and, in the case of residencies in the clinical divisions of medicine, surgery, and other special fields, advanced training in preparation for the practice of a specialty

Resident: 1. A common synonym for patient, especially in long-term care 2. A graduate physician in post-graduate hospital clinical training

Resident assessment instrument (RAI): A uniform assessment instrument developed by the Centers for Medicare and Medicaid Services to standardize the collection of skilled nursing facility patient data;

includes the Minimum Data Set 2.0, triggers, and resident assessment protocols; *See* **Minimum Data Set**

Resident assessment protocol (RAP): A summary of a long-term care resident's medical condition and care requirements

Resident Assessment Validation and Entry (RAVEN): A type of data-entry software developed by the Centers for Medicare and Medicaid Services for long-term care facilities and used to collect Minimum Data Set assessments and to transmit data to state databases

Resident care facility: A facility that provides accommodations, supervision, and personal care services for those who are dependent on services of others due to age or physical or mental impairment

Resident care facility for the elderly (RCFE): A residential facility that provides room, board, housekeeping, supervision, and personal care assistance for persons who are unable to live by themselves but who do not need 24-hour nursing care

Resident classification system: A system for classifying skilled nursing facility residents into mutually exclusive groups based on clinical, functional, and resource-based criteria

Residential arrangement: The situation in which an individual lives on a regular basis: owns a home or apartment; resides in a facility where health, disability, or aging-related services or supervision are available; resides in another residential setting where no services are provided; resides in a nursing home or other health facility; resides in another institutional setting such as a prison; is homeless or lives in a shelter for the homeless; lives in a place unknown or not stated

Residential care: Services, including board and lodging, provided in a protective environment but with minimal supervision to residents who are not in an acute phase of illness and would be capable of self-preservation during an emergency

Resident record: A term frequently used in long-term care in lieu of health record

Resident's right to access: A term encompassing the mechanisms in place to allow residents to review their own health information

Resource-based relative value scale (RBRVS): A Medicare reimbursement system implemented in 1992 to compensate physicians according to a fee schedule predicated on weights assigned on the basis of the resources required to provide the services

Resource intensity: The relative volume and types of diagnostic, therapeutic, and bed services used in the management of a particular illness

Resources: The labor, equipment, or materials needed to complete a project

Resource Utilization Groups, Version III (RUG-III): A case-mix–adjusted classification system based on Minimum Data Set assessments and used by skilled nursing facilities

Respect for Persons: The principle that all people are presumed to be free and responsible and should be treated accordingly

Respiratory therapy (RT): Services provided by a qualified professional for the assessment, treatment, and monitoring of patients with deficiencies or abnormalities of pulmonary function

Respite care: A type of short-term care provided during the day or overnight to individuals in the home or institution to temporarily relieve the family home caregiver

Responsibility: The accountability required as part of a job, such as supervising work performed by others or managing assets or funds

Responsibility center: A department as a whole, headed by an individual who is responsible for operations

Restitution: The act of returning something to its rightful owner, of making good or giving something equivalent for any loss, damage, or injury

Restorative nursing care: Care that incorporates resident-specific programs that restore and preserve function to assist the resident in maximizing functional independence and achieving a satisfactory quality of life

Restraints and seclusion: Ways of managing behavior; the right of patients to be free from non-medically necessary restraints and seclusion is protected under the Medicare Conditions of Participation

Restriction: Partially closing an orifice or the lumen of a tubular body part. Coded when the objective of the procedure is to narrow the diameter of a tubular body part or orifice in ICD-10-PCS

Resubmittal: The process of sending a corrected, or now complete, claim to an insurance company for reconsideration of the original payment or denial; *Also called* **rebill**

Results management: Results retrieval technology that permits viewing of data by type and manipulation of several different types of data. Also referred to as results management systems

Results retrieval: A lookup system that enables a user to access several different types of data from different source systems through a single application screen

Retained earnings: Undistributed profits from a for-profit organization that stay in the business

Retaliation and waiver: Rights protected under the Privacy Rule; to ensure the integrity of individuals' right to complain about alleged Privacy Rule violations, covered entities are expressly prohibited from retaliating against anyone who exercises his or her rights under the Privacy Rule, assists in an investigation by the HHS or other appropriate investigative authority, or opposes an act or practice that the person believes is a violation of the Privacy Rule. Individuals cannot be required to waive the rights that they hold under the Privacy Rule in order to obtain treatment, payment, or enrollment and benefits eligibility

Retention: 1. Mechanisms for storing records, providing for timely retrieval, and establishing the length of times that various types of records will be retained by the healthcare organization 2. The ability to keep valuable employees from seeking employment elsewhere

Retention policy: A policy that establishes how long the healthcare facility should keep health records, the medium in which the information will be kept, and where the records will be located and retrieved. Types of information retained may vary by state and accrediting body

Retention schedules: A time line for various records retention based on factors such as federal and state laws, statutes of limitations, age of patient, competency of patient, accreditation standards, AHIMA recommendations, and operational needs

Retinal detachment: The separation of two layers of the retina from each other, which usually occurs when the vitreous adheres to the retina (the sensitive layer of the eye) and "pulls," resulting in retinal holds that tear that may lead to retinal detachment

Retraction: The act of correcting information that was inaccurate, invalid, or made in error and preventing its display or hiding the entry or documentation from further view

Retrievability: Efficiently finding relevant information

Retrograde: Moving backward, against the normal flow

Retrospective: A type of time frame that looks back in time

Retrospective coding: A type of coding that takes place after the patient has been discharged and the entire health record has been routed to the health information management department

Retrospective payment method: *See* **retrospective payment system**

Retrospective payment system: Type of fee-for-service reimbursement in which providers receive recompense after health services have been rendered; *Also called* **retrospective payment method**

Retrospective review: The part of the utilization review process that concentrates on a review of clinical information following patient discharge

Retrospective study: A type of research conducted by reviewing records from the past (for example, birth and death certificates and/or health records) or by obtaining information about past events through surveys or interviews

Retrospective utilization review: A review of records some time after the patient's discharge or date of service to determine any of several issues, including the quality or appropriateness of the care provided

Return: The increase in value of an investment

Return on assets (ROA): The return on a company's investment, or earnings, after taxes divided by total assets

Return on equity (ROE): A more comprehensive measurement of profitability that takes into consideration the organization's net value

Return on investment (ROI): The financial analysis of the extent of value a major purchase will provide

Revenge effects: Unintended and typically negative consequences of a change in technology

Revenue: The charges generated from providing healthcare services; earned and measurable income

Revenue code: A three- or four-digit number in the chargemaster that totals all items and their charges for printing on the form used for Medicare billing

Revenue cycle: 1. The process of how patient financial and health information moves into, through, and out of the healthcare facility, culminating with the facility receiving reimbursement for services provided 2. The regularly repeating set of events that produces revenue

Revenue cycle management: The supervision of all administrative and clinical functions that contribute to the capture, management, and collection of patient service revenue, with the goals of accelerated cash flow and lowered accounts receivable

Revenues: The charges generated from providing healthcare services; earned and measurable income

Reverse mentoring: The opposite of the usual coaching process where the younger goes to the older instructor

Review of systems (ROS): A uniform system of performing an inventory of body systems through a series of questions seeking to identify signs and/or symptoms the patient may be experiencing or has experienced

Revision: 1. Correcting, to the extent possible, a malfunctioning or displaced device. Can include correcting a malfunctioning device by taking out and/or putting in part but not all of the device 2. Correction or alteration to the health record

Revocation: The act of withdrawing an authorization or permission that was previously granted as in the case of consents or authorizations to disclose information or requesting restrictions

Rewarding stage: In performance management, the fifth of five stages during which individual employees are rewarded for exceptional achievement

RFE: *See* **reasons for encounter**

RFI: *See* **request for information**

RFID: *See* **radio frequency identification**

RFP: *See* **request for proposal**

RHHI: *See* **regional home health intermediaries**

RHIA: *See* **registered health information administrator**

RHIN: *See* **regional health information network**

RHIO: *See* **regional health information organization**

RHIT: *See* **registered health information technician**

RIC: *See* **rehabilitation impairment category**

Rider: Document added to a healthcare insurance policy that provides details about coverage or lack of coverage for special situations that are not usually included in standard policies; may function as an exclusion or limitation

Right-to-work laws: Federal legislation dealing with labor rights (examples include workers' compensation, child labor, and minimum wage laws)

RIPA: *See* **radioimmunoprecipitation assay**

Rip-and-replace: An information technology acquisition strategy in which older technology is replaced with new technology

Risk: 1. The probability of incurring injury or loss 2. The probable amount of loss foreseen by an insurer in issuing a contract 3. A formal insurance term denoting liability to compensate individuals for injuries sustained in a healthcare facility

Risk adjustment: Any method of comparing the severity of illness of one group of patients with that of another group of patients; *See* **case-mix adjustment; severity-of-illness adjustment**

Risk analysis: The process of identifying possible security threats to the organization's data and identifying which risks should be proactively addressed and which risks are lower in priority; *Also called* risk assessment

Risk corridors: Established by the Medicare Prescription Drug, Improvement, and Modernization Act of 2003 for prescription drug plans and Medicare Advantage drug plans to help keep payments in line with actual costs while giving plans an incentive to control these costs

Risk evaluation: The final step in the risk management process, which involves evaluating each piece of the process in order to determine whether objectives are being met

Risk exposure or identification: A systematic means of identifying potential losses, which requires an understanding of the facility's business, legal, organizational, and clinical components

Risk financing: Methods used to pay for the costs associated with claims and other expenses; most commonly, liability insurance

Risk management (RM): A comprehensive program of activities intended to minimize the potential for injuries to occur in a facility and to anticipate and respond to ensuring liabilities for those injuries that do occur. The processes in place to identify, evaluate, and control risk, defined as the organization's risk of accidental financial liability

Risk of mortality (ROM): The likelihood of an inpatient death for a patient

Risk pool: Distribution of risk among a larger group of persons (insured). This group of persons have similar risks of loss

Risk prevention: One component of a successful risk management program

Risk sharing agreement: An agreement in which a vendor assumes at least part of the responsibility, from a financial perspective, for a successful computer system implementation

Risk–transfer mechanism: A mechanism whereby risk is passed from a regulated insurer to a quasi-regulated, regulated, or nonregulated provider

Risk treatment: The application of risk control and risk financing techniques to determine how a risk should be treated, often aimed at preventing or reducing the chances and/or effects of a loss occurrence

RLS: *See* **record locator service**

RM: *See* **risk management**

RMRS: *See* **Regenstrief medical records system**

RN: *See* **registered nurse**

R/O: Rule out

ROE: *See* **return on equity**

ROI: *See* **release of information; return on investment**

ROLAP: *See* **relational online analytical processing**

Role-based access control (RBAC): A control system in which access decisions are based on the roles of individual users as part of an organization

Role playing: A training method in which participants are required to respond to specific problems they may actually encounter in their jobs

Role theory: Thinking that attempts to explain how people adopt specific roles, including leadership roles

Roles and responsibilities: The definition of who does what on a project and the hierarchy for decision making

ROM: *See* **risk of mortality**

Root-cause analysis: A technique used in performance improvement initiatives to discover the underlying causes of a problem. Analysis of a sentinel event from all aspects (human, procedural, machinery, material) to identify how each contributed to the occurrence of the event and to develop new systems that will prevent recurrence

Root concept: A single special concept that represents the root of the entire content in SNOMED CT

Root operation: The third character of an ICD-10-PCS code that defines the objective of the procedure

ROS: *See* **review of systems**

Router: A device that attaches multiple networks and routes packets between the networks using software

Row/record: A set of columns or a collection of related data items in a table

RR: *See* **relative risk**

RT: *See* **respiratory therapy**

Rubric: A category; in ICPC, the two digits following the first character of an ICPC code and representing the second axis, components

RUG-III: *See* **Resource Utilization Groups, Version III**

Rule induction: *See* **association rule analysis**

Rules and regulations: Operating documents that describe the rules and regulations under which a healthcare organization operates; *See* **bylaws**

Rules engine: A computer program that applies sophisticated mathematical models to data that generate alerts and reminders to support healthcare decision making

Run chart: A type of graph that shows data points collected over time and identifies emerging trends or patterns

Rural area: Geographic area outside an urban area and its constituent counties or count equivalents. Any area not designated as a metropolitan statistical area for the purposes of case-mix index sets and wage index adjustments to federal Medicare reimbursement rates; *See* **core-based statistical area (CBSA); metropolitan statistical area (MSA)**

RVS: *See* **relative value scale**

RVU: *See* **relative value unit**

RW: *See* **relative weight**

RxNorm: A clinical drug nomenclature developed by the Food and Drug Administration, the Department of Veterans Affairs, and HL7 to provide standard names for clinical drugs and administered dose forms

SaaS: *See* **Software as a Service**

Safe practices: Behaviors undertaken to reduce or prevent adverse effects and medical errors

Safety management: A system for providing a risk-free environment for patients, visitors, and employees

Sample: A set of units selected for study that represents a population

Sample size: The number of subjects needed in a study to represent a population

Sample size calculation: The qualitative and quantitative procedures to determine an appropriate sample size

Sample survey: A type of survey that collects data from representative members of a population

SAN: *See* **storage area network**

Sanctions: Penalties or other methods of enforcement used to provide incentives for compliance with laws or rules and regulations such as the HIPAA Privacy and Security Rules and related policies and procedures of the covered entity; sanctions should be uniform across organizations

Satellite clinic: A primary care facility, owned and operated by a hospital or other organization, which is located in an area convenient to patients or close to a specific patient population

Satisficing: A decision-making process in which the decision maker accepts a solution to a problem that is satisfactory rather than optimal

Scalable: The measure of a system to grow relative to various measures of size, speed, number of users, volume of data, and so on

Scalar chain: A theory in the chain of command in which everyone is included and authority and responsibility flow downward from the top of the organization

Scale: Measure with progressive categories, such as size, amount, importance, rank, or agreement

Scales of measurement: A reference standard for data collection and classification; *See* **categorical data; interval level data; nominal level data; ordinal level data; ratio level data**

Scanning: The process by which a document is read into an optical imaging system

Scatter chart: *See* **scatter diagram**

Scatter diagram: A graph that visually displays the linear relationships among factors

Scattergram: *See* **scatter plot**

Scatter plot: A visual representation of data points on an interval or ratio level used to depict relationships between two variables; *See* **scatter diagram**; **scattergram**

SCD: *See* **semantic clinical drug**

SCDC: *See* **semantic clinical drug component**

Scenarios: Stories describing the current and feasible future states of the business environment

Scheduling engine: A specific functionality in project management software that automates the assignment of task start and finish dates and, as a result, the expected project finish date

SCHIP: *See* **State Children's Health Insurance Program**

SCIC adjustment: *See* **significant change in condition adjustment**

Scientific inquiry: A process that comprises making predictions, collecting and analyzing evidence, testing alternative theories, and choosing the best theory

Scientific management: A principle that states that the best management is a science based on laws and rules and that secures maximum prosperity for both employer and employee

Scope: A term used in project management. A scope is a detailed statement that outlines and describes all work necessary to complete a project

Scope creep: A process in which the scope of a project grows while the project is in process, virtually guaranteeing that it will be over budget and behind schedule

Scope of command: The number and type of employees who report to a specific management position in a defined organizational structure

Scope of work: A term used in project management. A document that sets forth requirements for performance of work to achieve the project objectives

Scorecards: Reports of outcomes measures to help leaders know what they have accomplished; *Also called* **dashboards**

SCP: *See* **standard cost profile**

Screening mammography: Breast imaging, usually done with two views bilaterally, to detect unsuspected cancer in an asymptomatic woman

Screen prototype: A sketch of the user interface of each screen that is anticipated in a project

SDLC: *See* **systems development life cycle**

SDM: *See* **Semantic Data Model**

SDO: *See* **standards development organization**

Search engine: A software program used to search for data in databases (for example, a structured query language)

SEC: *See* **Securities and Exchange Commission**

Secondary analysis: A method of research involving analysis of the original work of another person or organization

Secondary care: A general term for healthcare services provided by a specialist at the request of the primary care physician

Secondary data source: Data derived from the primary patient record, such as an index or a database

Secondary diagnosis: A statement of those conditions coexisting during a hospital episode that affect the treatment received or the length of stay

Secondary insurer: The insurance carrier that pays benefits after the primary payer has determined and paid its obligation

Secondary release of information: A type of information release in which the initial requester forwards confidential information to others without obtaining required patient authorization

Secondary research: Processing data that has already been collected by another party

Secondary source: A summary of an original work, such as an encyclopedia

Secondary storage: The permanent storage of data and programs on disks or tapes

Secondary variable: *See* **confounding variable**

Second opinion: Opinion obtained from a second physician regarding the necessity for a treatment that has been recommended by the first physician. Cost containment measure to prevent unnecessary tests, treatments, medical devices, or surgical procedures

Secure messaging system: A system that eliminates the security concerns that surround e-mail, but retains the benefits of proactive, traceable, and personalized messaging; *Also called* secure notification delivery system

Securities and Exchange Commission (SEC): The federal agency that regulates all public and some private transactions involving the ownership and debt of organizations

Security: 1. The means to control access and protect information from accidental or intentional disclosure to unauthorized persons and from unauthorized alteration, destruction, or loss 2. The physical protection of facilities and equipment from theft, damage, or unauthorized access; collectively, the policies, procedures, and safeguards designed to protect the confidentiality of information, maintain the integrity and availability of information systems, and control access to the content of these systems

Security audit process: A process put into place by a healthcare organization to monitor the effectiveness of its security program and to ensure compliance with it

Security breach: A violation of the policies or standards developed to ensure security

Security management: The oversight of facilities, equipment, and other resources, including human resources and technology, to reduce the possibility of harm to or theft of these assets of an organization

Security officer or chief security officer: The Security Rule mandates an individual to be in charge of the security program for the covered entity. HIPAA calls this individual a security official; however this position is frequently called chief security officer (CSO) by the covered entities. This person is responsible for overseeing privacy policies and procedures and managing the organization's information security program

Security program: A plan outlining the policies and procedures created to protect healthcare information

Security pyramid: A graphic representation of security measures in which each depends on the one below it

Security Rule: The federal regulations created to implement the security requirements of the Health Insurance Portability and Accountability Act of 1996

Security standards: Statements that describe the processes and procedures meant to ensure that patient-identifiable health information remains confidential and protected from unauthorized disclosure, alteration, and destruction

Security threat: A situation that has the potential to damage a healthcare organization's information system

Selection: The act or process of choosing

Selective catheter placement: Catheter placement into any arterial or venous vessel other than the aorta, vena cava, or the original vessel that was punctured

Self-directed learning: An instructional method that allows students to control their learning and progress at their own pace

Self-efficacy: Confidence in one's personal capabilities to do a job. The belief in one's capacity to organize and carry out a course of action to manage a situation

Self-insured plan: Method of insurance in which the employer or other association itself administers the health insurance benefits for its employees or their dependents, thereby assuming the risks for the costs of healthcare for the group

Self-monitoring: The act of observing the reactions of others to one's behavior and making the necessary behavioral adjustments to improve the reactions of others in the future

Self-pay: Type of fee-for-service reimbursement in which the patients or their guarantors pay a specific amount for each service received

Self-reported health status: A method of measuring health status in which a person rates his or her own general health, for example, by using a five-category classification: excellent, very good, good, fair, or poor

Semantic clinical drug (SCD): Standardized names created in RxNorm for every clinical drug; consists of components and a dose form

Semantic clinical drug component (SCDC): One of the two types of semantic normal forms created in RxNorm for every clinical drug, the SCDC consists of an active ingredient and strength

Semantic Clinical Drug (SCD) of RxNorm: *See* **semantic clinical drug**

Semantic Data Model (SDM): A natural application modeling mechanism that can capture and express the structure of an application environment; LOINC is an example of a semantic data model

Semantic differential scale: A measure that records a group's perception of a product, organization, or program through bipolar adjectives on a seven-point continuum, resulting in a profile

Semantic interoperability: Mutual understanding of the meaning of data exchanged between information systems

Semantic Network: The network that represents a consistent categorization of all concepts represented in the UMLS Metathesaurus

Semantic normal form (SNF): The preferred term for clinical drugs in RxNorm

Semantics: The meaning of a word or term; sometimes refers to comparable meaning, usually achieved through a standard vocabulary

Semicolon: A punctuation mark [;] placed after a procedure description within a CPT code set to avoid repeating common information

Semistructured question: A type of question that begins with a structured question and follows with an unstructured question to clarify

Sensitivity label: A security level associated with the content of the information

Sentinel event: According to the Joint Commission, an unexpected occurrence involving death or serious physical or psychological injury, or the risk thereof. Serious injury specifically includes loss of limb or function. The phrase "or risk thereof" includes any process variation for which a recurrence would carry a significant chance of serious adverse outcome. Such events are called "sentinel" because they signal the need for immediate investigation and response

Separate procedure: A procedure that is commonly part of another, more complex procedure, but which may be performed independently or be otherwise unrelated to the procedure

SEPs: Somatosensory evoked potentials

Sequence diagram: A systems analysis tool for documenting the interaction between an actor and the information system

Serial filing system: A health record identification system in which a patient receives sequential unique numerical identifiers for each encounter with, or admission to, a healthcare facility

Serial numbering system: A type of health record identification and filing system in which patients are assigned a different but unique numerical identifier for every admission

Serial–unit numbering system: A health record identification system in which patient numbers are assigned in a serial manner but records are brought forward and filed under the last number assigned

Server: A type of computer that makes it possible to share information resources across a network of client computers

Server redundancy: Situation where two servers are duplicating effort

Service: 1. An act performed by a person on behalf of another person 2. The means by which a defendant is notified of a lawsuit

Service bonus: A monetary reward given to long-term staff in recognition of their skills and commitment to the organization

Service Level Agreement (SLA): A contract between a customer and a service provider that records the common understanding about service priorities, responsibilities, guarantees, and other terms, especially related to availability, serviceability, performance, operation, or other attributes of the service like billing and penalties in the case of violation of the SLA

Service-line coder: A person who excels in coding one particular service line, such as oncology or cardiology

Service utilization domain: The range of available services including the patient's use of inpatient services preceding home care admission and the receipt of rehabilitation therapies during the home health episode

Severity indexing: 1. The process of using clinical evidence to identify the level of resource consumption 2. A method for determining degrees of illness

Severity of illness (SI or SOI): A type of supportive documentation reflecting objective clinical indicators of a patient illness (essentially the patient is sick enough to be at an identified level of care) and referring to the extent of physiologic decompensation or organ system loss of function

Severity of illness adjustment: *See* **risk adjustment**

Severity-of-illness (SI) screening criteria: Standards used to determine the most appropriate setting of care based on the level of clinical signs and symptoms that a patient shows upon presentation to a healthcare facility

Severity-of-illness system: A database established from coded data on diseases and operations and used in the hospital for planning and research purposes

Severity weight (SW): A factor developed by 3M to indicate relative severity within every level in APR-DRGs and used to improve comparisons in profiling by severity-adjusted raw statistics

SF: Straightforward

SGML: *See* **standard generalized markup language**

Shared systems: Systems developed by data-processing companies in the 1960s and 1970s to address the computing needs of healthcare organizations that could not afford, or chose not to purchase, their own mainframe computing systems

Shared Visions—New Pathways: The new accreditation process implemented by the Joint Commission in January 2004 and designed to focus on systems critical to the safety and quality of patient care, treatment, and services

Shareware: A type of software that can be tried before being purchased

Shaving: The sharp removal, by transverse incision or horizontal slicing, of epidermal and superficial dermal lesions without a full-thickness dermal excision; includes local anesthesia and chemical or electrocauterization of the wound; wound does not require suture closure

Sheltered employment: An employment category provided in a special industry or workshop for the physically, mentally, emotionally, or developmentally handicapped

Shift differential: An increased wage paid to employees who work less desirable shifts, such as evenings, nights, or weekends

Shift rotation: The assignment of employees to different periods of service to provide coverage, as needed

Short-stay outlier: Hospitalization that is five-sixths of the geometric length of stay for the long-term care diagnosis related group (LTC-DRG)

Short-stay patient: A patient admitted to the hospital for an intended stay of less than 24 hours and who is considered an outpatient and not included in inpatient hospital census statistics

SI: *See* **severity of illness**

Signal tracing data: *See* **vector graphic data**

Significance level: The criterion used for rejecting the null hypothesis; a preestablished cutoff that determines whether the null hypothesis is rejected; the alpha level

Significant change in condition (SCIC) adjustment: A single episode payment under multiple home health resource groups, each prorated to the number of service days delivered

Significant procedure: A procedure that is surgical in nature or carries a procedural or an anesthetic risk or requires specialized training

Significant procedure ambulatory payment classification: A procedure that constitutes the reason for the visit, dominates the time and resources rendered during the visit, and is not subject to payment reduction or discounting

Sign-on bonus: A monetary incentive used by a facility to encourage a candidate to accept employment

Simon's decision-making model: A model proposing that the decision-making process moves through three phases: intelligence, design, and choice

Simple complete mastectomy: The removal of all of the breast tissue without removing lymph nodes or muscles

Simple payback method: A method used to justify a proposed capital expenditure where the asset cost is divided by the net annual income of the asset to determine how long it will take for the asset to "pay back" what it cost the organization

Simple random sampling: The process of selecting units from a population so that each one has exactly the same chance of being included in the sample

Simulation: A training technique for experimenting with real-world situations by means of a computerized model that represents the actual situation

Simulation and inventory modeling: The key components of a plan that are computer simulated for testing and experimentation so that optimal operational procedures can be found

Simulation observation: A type of nonparticipant observation in which researchers stage events rather than allowing them to happen naturally

Simultaneous equations method: A budgeting concept that distributes overhead costs through multiple iterations, allowing maximum distribution of interdepartmental costs among overhead departments

Single-blinded study: A study design in which (typically) the investigator but not the subject knows the identity of the treatment and control groups

Single sign-on: A type of technology that allows a user access to all disparate applications through one authentication procedure, thus reducing the number and variety of passwords a user must remember and enforcing and centralizing access control

Site visit: An in-person review conducted by an accreditation survey team; the visit involves document reviews, staff interviews, an examination of the organization's physical plant, and other activities

Six Sigma: Disciplined and data-driven methodology for getting rid of defects in any process

Sixty-day episode payment: The basic unit of payment under the home health prospective payment system that covers a beneficiary for 60 days regardless of the number of days furnished unless the beneficiary elects to transfer, has a significant change in condition, or is discharged and then returns to the same agency within the 60-day episode

Skewness: The horizontal stretching of a frequency distribution to one side or the other so that one tail is longer than the other, creating a negative or positive skew

Skill: The ability, education, experience, and training required to perform a job task

Skilled nursing facility (SNF): A long-term care facility with an organized professional staff and permanent facilities (including inpatient beds) that provides continuous nursing and other health-related, psychosocial, and personal services to patients who are not in an acute phase of illness but who primarily require continued care on an inpatient basis

Skilled nursing facility prospective payment system (SNF PPS): A per-diem reimbursement system implemented in July 1998 for costs (routine, ancillary, and capital) associated with covered skilled nursing facility services furnished to Medicare Part A beneficiaries

Skin graft: Skin tissue that is completely detached from its blood supply in the donor area and reattached to a blood supply from the base of the wound or the recipient area

Sliding scale: A method of billing in which the cost of healthcare services is based on the patient's income and ability to pay

SLMBs: *See* **specified low-income Medicare beneficiaries**

SLP: *See* **speech-language therapy**

Smart card: A credit card–sized piece of plastic embedded with a computer chip that stores information and incorporates security features

SMI: *See* **supplemental medical insurance** (Medicare Part B)

SNF: *See* **semantic normal form; skilled nursing facility**

SNF market basket index: *See* **skilled nursing facility market basket index**

SNF PPS: *See* **skilled nursing facility prospective payment system**

Sniffers: A software security product that runs in the background of a network, examining and logging packet traffic and serving as an early warning device against crackers

SNODENT: *See* **Systematized Nomenclature of Dentistry**

SNOMED: *See* **Systemized Nomenclature of Human and Veterinary Medicine**

SNOMED CT: *See* **Systemized Nomenclature of Medicine Clinical Terminology**

SNOMED RT: *See* **Systemized Nomenclature of Medicine Reference Terminology**

Snowflake schema: A modification of the star schema in which the dimension tables are further divided to reduce data redundancy. Used in data warehouses

SOAP: An acronym for a component of the problem-oriented medical record that refers to how each progress note contains documentation relative to **s**ubjective observations, **o**bjective observations, **a**ssessments, and **p**lans

SOAPIER: A form of charting narrative notes that requires **s**ubjective, **o**bjective, **a**ssessment, **p**lan, **i**ntervention, **e**valuation, and **r**evision in the note structure

Socialization: The process of influencing the behavior and attitudes of a new employee to adapt positively to the work environment

Social Security Act of 1935: The federal legislation that originally established the Social Security program as well as unemployment compensation and support for mothers and children; amended in 1965 to create the Medicare and Medicaid programs

Social Security number (SSN): A unique numerical identifier assigned to every US citizen

SOF: Signature on file

Software: A program that directs the hardware components of a computer system to perform the tasks required

Software as a Service (SaaS): Software that is provided through an outsourcing contract and is deployed over the Internet

SOI: *See* **severity of illness**

Sole-community hospital: Hospital that, by reason of factors such as isolated location, weather conditions, travel conditions, or absence of other hospitals (as determined by the Secretary of the Department of Health and Human Services [HHS]), is the sole source of patient hospital services reasonably available to individuals in a geographical area who are entitled to benefits

Sole proprietorship: A venture with one owner in which all profits are considered the owner's personal income

Solo practice: A practice in which the physician is self-employed and legally the sole owner

Solvency: The state of being able to pay all debts

Sound data: *See* **real audio data**

Source of admission: The point from which a patient enters a healthcare organization, including physician referral, clinic referral, health maintenance organization referral, transfer from a hospital, transfer from a skilled nursing facility, transfer from another healthcare facility, emergency department referral, court or law enforcement referral, and delivery of newborns

Source of admission code: Required code for Medicare that indicates the admission source

Source of truth: The official source of information that will be used for legal purposes for a particular request for information

Source-oriented health record format: A system of health record organization in which information is arranged according to the patient care department that provided the care

Source system: 1. A system in which data was originally created 2. Independent information system application that contributes data to an EHR, including departmental clinical applications (for example, laboratory information system, clinical pharmacy information system)

and specialty clinical applications (for example, intensive care, cardiology, labor and delivery)

Spaced training: The process of learning a task in sections separated by time

Span of control: Concept of classical organization theory that suggests managers are capable of supervising only a limited number of employees

Special care unit: A medical care unit in which there is appropriate equipment and a concentration of physicians, nurses, and others who have special skills and experience to provide optimal medical care for critically ill patients or continuous care of patients in special diagnostic categories

Special-cause variation: An unusual source of variation that occurs outside a process but affects it

SPECIALIST Lexicon: A tool that supplies the lexical information needed for the SPECIALIST natural language processing (NLP) system

Specialty software: A type of applications software that performs specialized, niche functions such as encoding or drawing and painting

Specified low-income Medicare beneficiaries (SLMBs): Medicare beneficiaries who have resources similar to qualified Medicare beneficiaries, but higher incomes, although still less than 120 percent of the federal poverty level

Specimen: Tissue submitted for individual and separate attention, requiring individual examination and pathologic diagnosis

Speech-language therapy (SLP): A treatment intended to improve or enhance the resident's ability to communicate and/or swallow

Speech recognition: Situation where speech is converted to text on a screen

Speech recognition technology: Technology that translates speech to text

Spin-off: A new, separate company formed by a parent company and whose shares are distributed to existing shareholders of the parent company in proportion to the new entity's relationship to the parent company

Spirometry: The measurement of the breathing capacity of the lungs

SPL: *See* **Clinical Special Product Label**

Split percentage payment: A type of reimbursement in which payments are made for each episode period, and home health agencies receive two payments to make up the total permissible reimbursement for the episode

Splitter vocabulary: A type of vocabulary that permits storage of each concept in a sample narrative. SNOMED is an example of a splitter vocabulary

Sponsor: A person or an entity that initiates a clinical investigation of a drug (usually the drug manufacturer or research institution that developed the drug) by distributing it to investigators for clinical trials; a person in an organization that supports, protects, and promotes an idea within the organization; the company position with the ultimate responsibility for a project's success

SQL: *See* **structured query language**

SSA: Social Security Administration

SSN: *See* **Social Security number**

Stable monetary unit: The currency used as the measurement of financial transactions

Staff authority: The lines of reporting in the organizational chart in which the position advises or makes recommendations

Staffing analysis: Study performed to determine the most efficient and cost-effective staff mix

Staffing structure: The arrangement of staff positions within an organization

Staff model health maintenance organization: A type of health maintenance that employs physicians to provide healthcare services to subscribers; *See* **closed panel**

Staff retention: The process of keeping valued employees on the job and reducing turnover

Stage of the neoplasm: A classification of malignancies (cancers) according to the anatomic extent of the tumor, such as primary neoplasm, regional lymph nodes, and metastases

Stages of grief: A five-stage model created by Kübler-Ross describing how people progress through loss to acceptance in response to death that may be applied to similar changes experienced by employees in response to organizational transition. The five stages are: shock and denial, anger, bargaining, depression, and acceptance

Staging system: A method used in cancer registers to identify specific and separate different stages or aspects of the disease

Stakeholder: An individual within the company who has an interest in, or is affected by, the results of a project

Standard: 1. A scientifically based statement of expected behavior against which structures, processes, and outcomes can be measured 2. A model or example established by authority, custom, or general consent or a rule established by an authority as a measure of quantity, weight, extent, value, or quality

Standard cost profile (SCP): A set of data that identifies, analyzes, and defines the activities, including the costs, of departments within the organization to produce a service unit

Standard deviation: A measure of variability that describes the deviation from the mean of a frequency distribution in the original units of measurement; the square root of the variance

Standard federal rate: National base payment amount in the prospective payment system for long-term care hospitals (PPS for LTC). This amount is multiplied with the relative weight of the long-term care diagnosis-related group (LTC-DRG) to calculate the unadjusted payment. Published annually in the *Federal Register.*

Standard generalized markup language (SGML): An International Standards Organization standard that establishes rules for identifying elements within a text document

Standardized payment: National base amount in the inpatient rehabilitation facility prospective payment system (IRF PPS). This amount is multiplied with the relative weight of the case-mix group to calculate the unadjusted payment; published annually in the *Federal Register*

Standard normal distribution: Most of the values in a set of data are close to the "average" and relatively few values tend to one extreme or the other, creating a bell-shaped curve; *See* **normal distribution**

Standard of care: An established set of clinical decisions and actions taken by clinicians and other representatives of healthcare organizations in accordance with state and federal laws, regulations, and guidelines; codes of ethics published by professional associations or societies; regulations for accreditation published by accreditation agencies; usual and common practice of equivalent clinicians or organizations in a geographical region

Standard risk: A person who, according to an insured's underwriting standards, is entitled to purchase insurance without paying an extra premium or incurring special restrictions

Standards development organization (SDO): A private or government agency involved in the development of healthcare informatics standards at a national or international level

Standards for privacy of individually identifiable health information: *See* **Privacy Rule**

Standard treatment protocols (STPs): Protocols that identify the specific service units necessary to produce a given product (patient)

Standard vocabulary: A vocabulary that is accepted throughout the healthcare industry

Standing committees: Committees that are put in place to oversee ongoing and cross-functional issues (examples include the medical staff committee, a quality improvement committee, or an infection control committee)

Standing orders: Orders the medical staff or an individual physician has established as routine care for a specific diagnosis or procedure

Star schema: A visual method of expressing a multidimensional data structure in a relational database

State Children's Health Insurance Program (SCHIP): The children's healthcare program implemented as part of the Balanced Budget Act of 1997; sometimes referred to as the Children's Health Insurance Program, or CHIP

Statement: A list of unpaid invoices; sometimes a cumulative list of all transactions between purchaser and vendor during a specific time period

Statement of cash flow: A statement detailing the reasons why cash amounts changed from one balance sheet period to another; *Also called* **statement of changes in financial position**

Statement of changes in financial position: *See* **statement of cash flow**

Statement of changes in net assets: The accounting statement that explains the differences in net assets from period to period on the balance sheet

Statement of fund balance: *See* **statement of stockholder's equity**

Statement of operations: *See* **statement of revenue and expenses**

Statement of retained earnings: A statement expressing the change in retained earnings from the beginning of the balance sheet period to the end

Statement of revenue and expenses: A financial statement showing how much the organization makes or loses during a given reporting period; *Also called* **earnings report**; **income statement**; **profit and loss statement**; **statement of operations**

Statement of stockholder's equity: A statement detailing the reasons for changes in each stockholder's equity accounts; *Also called* **statement of fund balance**

Statement of work (SOW): A document that defines the scope and goals of a specific project; *Also called* **project charter**

State workers' compensation insurance funds: Funds that provide a stable source of insurance coverage for work-related illnesses and injuries and serve to protect employers from underwriting uncertainties by making it possible to have continuing availability of workers' compensation coverage

Statistical process control chart: A type of run chart that includes both upper and lower control limits and indicates whether a process is stable or unstable

Statistical inference: Helps to make inference or guess about a larger group of data by drawing conclusions from a small group of data

Statistical significance: The probability that an observed difference is due to chance

Statistics: A branch of mathematics concerned with collecting, organizing, summarizing, and analyzing data

Statute: A piece of legislation written and approved by a state or federal legislature and then signed into law by the state's governor or the president

Statute of limitations: A specific time frame allowed by a statute or law for bringing litigation

Statutory law: Written law established by federal and state legislatures; *Also called* **legislative law**

Stay outliers: *See* **outlier**

Stealth virus: A type of computer virus that attempts to hide itself by concealing its presence in infected files

Stem and leaf plot: A visual display that organizes data to show its shape and distribution, using two columns with the stem in the left-hand column and all leaves associated with that stem in the right-hand column; the "leaf" is the ones digit of the number, and the other digits form the "stem"

Step-down allocation: A budgeting concept in which overhead costs are distributed once, beginning with the area that provides the least amount of non-revenue-producing services

Step-down unit: A unit used for cardiac patients for care between the cardiac intensive care unit and a general medical or surgical unit

Stillbirth: The birth of a fetus, regardless of gestational age, that shows no evidence of life (such as heartbeats or respirations) after complete expulsion or extraction from the mother during childbirth

Stimulus: *See* **American Recovery and Reinvestment Act of 2009**

Stop-loss benefit: Specific amount, in a certain time frame such as one year, beyond which all covered healthcare services for that policyholder or dependent are paid at 100 percent by the healthcare insurance plan; *See* **catastrophic expense limit; maximum out-of-pocket cost**

Stop-loss insurance: A form of reinsurance that provides protection for medical expenses above a certain limit

Storage and retrieval: A healthcare facility's method for safely and securely maintaining and archiving individual patient health records for future reference

Storage area network (SAN): Storage devices organized into a network so that they can be accessible from any server in the network

Storage management software: Software used to manage the SAN, keep track of where data are stored, and move older data to less expensive, but still accessible, storage locations

Storming: The second of four steps that occur when creating a functional team, storming occurs when individual team members examine their role within the group

Storyboard: A graphic display tool used to communicate the details of performance improvement activities; a type of poster that includes text and graphics to describe and illustrate the activities of a PI project

Storytelling: A group process technique in which group members create stories describing the plausible future state of the business environment

STPs: *See* **special treatment procedures; standard treatment protocols**

Straight numeric filing system: A health record filing system in which health records are arranged in ascending numerical order

Strategic communications: Programs created to advance specific organizational goals such as promoting a new center or service, establishing a new program, or positioning the organization as a center of excellence in a specific discipline such as cardiology or oncology

Strategic decision making: A type of decision making that is usually limited to individuals, such as boards of directors, chief executive officers, and top-level executives, who make decisions about the healthcare organization's strategic direction

Strategic decision support system: *See* **decision support system (DSS)**

Strategic goals: Long-term objectives set by an organization to improve its operations

Strategic information systems (IS) planning: A process for setting IS priorities within an organization; the process of identifying and prioritizing IS needs based on the organization's strategic goals with the intent of ensuring that all IS technology initiatives are integrated and aligned with the organization's overall strategic plan

Strategic issue: A question, topic, opportunity, or concern that is addressed through strategic management

Strategic management: The art and science of formulating, implementing, and evaluating cross-functional decisions that enable an organization to achieve its objectives

Strategic plan: The document in which the leadership of a healthcare organization identifies the organization's overall mission, vision, and goals to help set the long-term direction of the organization as a business entity

Strategic planning: A disciplined effort to produce fundamental decisions that shape and guide what an organization is, what it does, and why it does it

Strategy: A course of action designed to produce a desired (business) outcome

Strategy map: A visual representation of the cause-and-effect relationships among the components of an organization's strategy

Stratified random sampling: The process of selecting the same percentages of subjects for a study sample as they exist in the subgroups (strata) of the population

Streaming video: *See* **motion video**

Stress testing: Testing performed toward the end of EHR implementation to ensure that the actual number, or load, of transactions that would be performed during peak hours can be performed

Structure: 1. A term from Donabedian's model of quality assessment that assesses an organization's ability to provide services in terms of both the physical building and equipment and the people providing the healthcare services 2. The foundations of caregiving, which include buildings, equipment, technologies, professional staff, and appropriate policies

Structure and content standards: Common data elements and definitions of the data elements to be included in an electronic patient record

Structured analysis: A pattern identification analysis performed for a specific task

Structured brainstorming: A group problem-solving technique wherein the team leader asks each participant to generate a list of ideas for the topic under discussion and then report them to the group in a nonjudgmental manner

Structured data: Binary, computer-readable data

Structured data entry: A type of healthcare data documentation about an individual using a controlled vocabulary rather than narrative text; *Also called* **discrete data**

Structured decision: A decision made by following a formula or a step-by-step process

Structured input (SI): Information that has been organized to allow identification and separation of the context of the information from its content

Structured interview: An interview format that uses a set of standardized questions that are asked of all applicants

Structured query language (SQL): A fourth-generation computer language that includes both DDL and DML components and is used to create and manipulate relational databases

Structured question: Close-ended question, which is used more for self-assessments, web-based or e-mailed surveys, or mailed and faxed surveys; *Also called* **closed-ended question**

Structure indicators: Quality indicators that measure the attributes of an organizational setting, such as number and qualifications of staff, adequacy of equipment and facilities, and adequacy of organizational policies and procedures

Structure measures: Indicators that measure the attributes of the healthcare setting (for example, adequacy of equipment and supplies)

Student membership: AHIMA membership category for students enrolled in an AHIMA-accredited or approved program

Subacute care: A type of step-down care provided after a patient is released from an acute care hospital (including nursing homes and other facilities that provide medical care, but not surgical or emergency care)

Subcutaneous mastectomy: The removal of breast tissue, leaving the skin of the breast and nipple intact. This type of mastectomy usually requires that a breast implant be inserted

Subject matter jurisdiction: Pertaining to district courts, jurisdiction to hear cases involving felonies and misdemeanors that fall under federal statutes

Subpoena: A command to appear at a certain time and place to give testimony on a certain matter; *Also called* **subpoena ad testificandum**

Subpoena ad testificandum: *See* **subpoena**

Subpoena duces tecum: A written order commanding a person to appear, give testimony, and bring all documents, papers, books, and records described in the subpoena. The devices are used to obtain documents during pretrial discovery and to obtain testimony during trial

Subpoena policy: A policy that outlines the steps required to handle subpoenas and e-discovery requests

Subprojects: Smaller components of a larger project

Subrogation: The means by which an insurance company recovers moneys from a third party; that amount paid to or on behalf of an insurer, usually sought in respect to a loss (for example, an accident or injury)

Subscriber: Individual or entity that purchases healthcare insurance coverage; *See* **certificate holder; insured; member; policyholder**

Substance Abuse and Mental Health Services Administration (SAMHSA): A division of the Department of Health and Human Services which in 2004 published a document explaining the relationship between HIPAA and the Alcohol and Drug Abuse Regulations regarding confidentiality and release of information

Successor: A task in a dependency relationship between two tasks that is dependent on the predecessor task

Summary list: *See* **problem list**

Summons: An instrument used to begin a civil action or special proceeding and is a means of acquiring jurisdiction over a party

Superbill: The office form used for physician office billing that is initiated by the physician and states the diagnoses and other information for each patient encounter

Supercomputer: The largest, fastest, and most expensive type of computer that exists today

Supervisory management: Management level that oversees the organization's efforts at the staff level and monitors the effectiveness of everyday operations and individual performance against preestablished standards

Supervisory managers: Managers who oversee small (2- to 10-person) functional workgroups or teams and often perform hands-on functions in addition to supervisory functions

Supplement: Putting in or on biological or synthetic material that physically reinforces and/or augments the function of a portion of a body part. The body part may have been taken out during a previous procedure, but is not taken out as part of the supplement procedure

Supplemental medical insurance (SMI): A small independent insurance policy that consumers may take out independently of their primary insurance that helps pay for physicians' services, medical services, and supplies not covered by Medicare Part A

Supply management: Management and control of the supplies used within an organization

Supreme Court: The highest court in the US legal system; hears cases from the US Courts of Appeals and the highest state courts when federal statutes, treaties, or the US Constitution is involved

Surgery: An umbrella term referring to the procedures of incision, excision, amputation, introduction, endoscopy, suture, and manipulation

Surgical death rate: *See* **postoperative death rate**

Surgical operation: One or more surgical procedures performed at one time for one patient via a common approach or for a common purpose

Surgical package: A global package for surgical procedures that refers to the payment policy of bundling payment for the various services associated with a surgery into a single payment covering professional services for preoperative care, the surgery itself, and postoperative care; *Also called* **global package**

Surgical procedure: Any single, separate, systematic process upon or within the body that can be complete in itself; is normally performed by a physician, dentist, or other licensed practitioner; can be performed either with or without instruments; and is performed to restore disunited or deficient parts, remove diseased or injured tissues, extract foreign matter, assist in obstetrical delivery, or aid in diagnosis

Surgical review: Evaluation of operative and other procedures, invasive and noninvasive, using the Joint Commission guidelines

Surgical specialties: A group of clinical specialties that concentrates on the provision of surgical services by physicians who have received advanced training in obstetrics and gynecology, ophthalmology, orthopedics, cardiovascular surgery, otorhinolaryngology, trauma surgery, neurosurgery, thoracic surgery, urology, plastic and reconstructive surgery, anesthesiology, and pathology

Survey: A method of self-report research in which the individuals themselves are the source of the data

Survey feedback: An organizational development technique in which data on practices and attitudes are gathered and participants interpret them in order to plan change

Survey team: A group of individuals sent by an accrediting agency (usually the Joint Commission) to review a healthcare organization for accreditation purposes

Survey tools: Research instruments that are used to gather data and information from respondents in a uniform manner through the administration of a predefined and structured set of questions and possible responses

SW: *See* **severity weight**

Swing beds: Hospital-based acute care beds that may be used flexibly to serve as acute or skilled nursing care

Synchronous: Occurring at the same time

Synergy: The interaction of parts to produce a greater outcome than would be obtained by the parts acting separately

Syntax: A term that refers to the comparable structure or format of data, usually as they are being transmitted from one system to another

System: A set of related and highly interdependent components that are operating for a particular purpose

Systematic literature review: Methodical approach to literature review that reduces the possibility of bias; characterized by explicit search criteria to identify literature, and inclusion and exclusion criteria to select articles and information sources, and evaluation against consistent methodological standards; *See* **integrative review; meta-analysis**

Systematic sampling: The process of selecting a sample of subjects for a study by drawing every *n*th unit on a list

Systematized Nomenclature of Dentistry (SNODENT): A systemized nomenclature of dentistry containing dental diagnoses, signs, symptoms, and complaints

Systematized Nomenclature of Human and Veterinary Medicine (SNOMED): A comprehensive clinical vocabulary developed by the College of American Pathologists, which is the most promising set of clinical terms available for a controlled vocabulary for healthcare

Systematized Nomenclature of Medicine Clinical Terminology (SNOMED CT): A concept-based terminology consisting of more than 110,000 concepts with linkages to more than 180,000 terms with unique computer-readable codes

System build: The creation of data dictionaries, tables, decision support rules, templates for data entry, screen layouts, and reports used in a system

System catalog: An integrated data dictionary (which is a component of a database management system) that generally contains information on data tables and relationships in addition to data definitions

System design: The second phase of the systems development life cycle

System implementation: The third phase of the systems development life cycle

System infectors: Computer viruses that infect the system areas of diskettes or the hard drive of a computer; *See* **boot-record infectors**

System maintenance and evaluation: The final phase of the systems development life cycle

System planning and analysis: The first phase of the systems development life cycle

Systems: The foundations of caregiving, which include buildings (environmental services), equipment (technical services), professional staff (human resources), and appropriate policies (administrative)

Systems analysis: Process of studying organizational operations and determining information systems requirements for a given application

Systems analyst: An individual who investigates, analyzes, designs, develops, installs, evaluates, and maintains an organization's healthcare information systems; is typically involved in all aspects of the systems development life cycle; and serves as a liaison among end users and programmers, database administrators, and other technical personnel; *Also called* **clinical systems analyst**

Systems development life cycle (SDLC): A model used to represent the ongoing process of developing (or purchasing) information systems

Systems theory: An interdisciplinary field of study that analyzes and describes how any group of objects work together to produce a result

Systems thinking: An objective way of looking at work-related ideas and processes with the goal of allowing people to uncover ineffective patterns of behavior and thinking and then finding ways to make lasting improvements

System testing: A type of testing performed by an independent organization to identify problems in information systems

Table: An organized arrangement of data, usually in columns and rows

Table of allowances: *See* **fee schedule**

Tacit knowledge: The actions, experiences, ideals, values, and emotions of an individual that tend to be highly personal and difficult to communicate (for example, corporate culture, organizational politics, and professional experience)

Tactic: A method for accomplishing an end

Tactical decision making: A type of decision making that usually affects departments or business units (and sometimes policies and procedures) and includes short- and medium-range plans, schedules, and budgets

Tactical plan: A strategic plan at the level of divisions and departments

TANF: *See* **temporary assistance for needy families**

Target population: A large group of individuals who are the focus of a study

Task: The step to be performed in order to complete a project or part of a project

Task analysis: A procedure for determining the specific duties and skills required of a job

Tax Equity and Fiscal Responsibility Act of 1982 (TEFRA): The federal legislation that modified Medicare's retrospective reimbursement system for inpatient hospital stays by requiring implementation of diagnosis-related groups and the acute care prospective payment system

Taxonomy: The principles of a classification system, such as data classification, and the study of the general principles of scientific classification

TC: *See* **technical component**

TCP/IP: *See* **transmission control protocol/Internet protocol**

TCS: Transaction and code sets

Teaching hospital: Hospital engaged in an approved graduate medical education residency program in medicine, osteopathy, dentistry, or podiatry

Team building: The process of organizing and acquainting a team and building skills for dealing with later team processes

Team charter: A document that explains the issues the team was initiated to address, describes the team's goal or vision, and lists the initial members of the team and their respective departments

Team facilitator: A PI team role primarily responsible for ensuring that an effective performance improvement process occurs by serving as advisor and consultant to the PI team; remaining a neutral, nonvoting member; suggesting alternative PI methods and procedures to keep the team on target and moving forward; managing group dynamics, resolving conflict, and modeling compromise; acting as coach and motivator for the team; assisting in consensus building when necessary; and recognizing team and individual achievements

Team group dynamics: Models of team development uniformly define four stages of progression in team group dynamics: cautious affiliation, competitiveness, harmonious cohesiveness, and collaborative teamwork

Team leader: A performance improvement team role responsible for championing the effectiveness of performance improvement activities in meeting customers' needs and for the content of a team's work

Team member: A performance improvement team role responsible for participating in team decision making and plan development; identifying opportunities for improvement; gathering, prioritizing, and analyzing data; and sharing knowledge, information, and data that pertain to the process under study

Team norms: The rules, both explicit and implied, that determine both acceptable and unacceptable behavior for a group

Team recorder/scribe: A performance improvement team role responsible for maintaining the records of a team's work during meetings, including any documentation required by the organization

Technical component (TC): The portion of radiological and other procedures that is facility based or nonphysician based (for example, radiology films, equipment, overhead, endoscopic suites, and so on)

Technical safeguard provisions: Five broad categories of controls that can be implemented from a technical standpoint using computer software: access controls, audit controls, data integrity, person or entity authentication, and transmission security

Technical skills: One of the three managerial skill categories, related to knowledge of the technical aspects of the business

Technology management: The planning and implementation of technological resources, as needed, to effectively and efficiently carry out the organization's mission

Technology push: 1. The view of information technology as being able to push organizations into new business areas 2. Technology where certain data are pushed or delivered to a particular computer

TEFRA: *See* **Tax Equity and Fiscal Responsibility Act of 1982**

Telecommunications: Voice and data communications

Telecommuting: A work arrangement in which at least a portion of the employee's work hours is spent outside the office (usually in the home) and the work is transmitted back to the employer via electronic means; *See* **telestaffing**

Telehealth: A telecommunications system that links healthcare organizations and patients from diverse geographic locations and transmits text and images for (medical) consultation and treatment; *Also called* **telemedicine**

Telematics: The use of telecommunications and networks to share information among a patient and healthcare providers located in different locations or sites

Telemedicine: A telecommunications system that links healthcare organizations and patients from diverse geographic locations and transmits text and images for (medical) consultation and treatment; *Also called* **telehealth**

Telephone callback procedures: Procedures used primarily when employees have access to an organization's health information systems from a remote location that verify whether the caller's number is authorized and prevent access when it is not

Telestaffing: *See* **telecommuting**

Telesurgery: The use of robotics to perform surgery. This allows surgery to be performed on a patient in a different location

Template: A pattern used in computer-based patient records to capture data in a structured manner

Template-based entry: A cross between free text and structured data entry. The user is able to pick and choose data that are entered frequently, thus requiring the entry of data that change from patient to patient

Temporary assistance for needy families (TANF): A federal program that provides states with grants to be spent on time-limited cash assistance for low-income families, generally limiting a family's lifetime cash welfare benefits to a maximum of five years and permitting states to impose other requirements; replaced the Aid to Families with Dependent Children program

Temporary budget variance: The difference between the budgeted and actual amounts of a line item that is expected to reverse itself in a subsequent period; the timing difference between the budget and the actual event

Temporary employee: A person who is employed for a temporary, definite period of time, such as to complete a specific project or to fill in for a permanent employee on vacation or other leave; or a person who is employed for an indefinite period of time but who receives none of the fringe benefits offered to permanent employees

Temporary National Codes: Codes established by insurers when a code is needed before the next January 1 annual update for permanent national codes; these codes are independent of the permanent national codes

Temporary privileges: Privileges granted for a limited time period to a licensed, independent practitioner on the basis of recommendations made by the appropriate clinical department or the president of the medical staff

Ten-step monitoring and evaluation process: The systematic and ongoing collection, organization, and evaluation of data related to indicator development promoted by the Joint Commission in the mid-1980s

Terminal: A term used to describe the hardware in a mainframe computer system by which data may be entered or retrieved

Terminal-digit filing system: A system of health record identification and filing in which the last digit or group of digits (terminal digits) in the health record number determines file placement

Termination: The act of ending something (for example, a job)

Termination of access: An administrative safeguard that is used when an employee changes job position, job roles or duties, or terminates employment with the organization

Termination process: A HIPAA-mandated process that terminates an employee's access immediately upon separation from the facility

Terminology: A set of terms representing the system of concepts of a particular subject field; a clinical terminology provides the proper use of clinical words as names or symbols

Terminology asset manager: This position develops data sets, nomenclatures, and classification standards, and in order to do so the HIM professional must understand the data needs of all stakeholders

Terminology standard: A terminology adopted by the appropriate standards-setting organizations for use in healthcare

Term neonate: Any neonate whose birth occurs from the beginning of the first day (267th day) of the 39th week through the end of the last day of the 42nd week (294th day), following onset of the last menstrual period

Term type (TTY): Each element of the normalized term in RxNorm

Tertiary care: Care centered on the provision of highly specialized and technologically advanced diagnostic and therapeutic services in inpatient and outpatient hospital settings

Testing: The act of performing an examination or evaluation

Test statistics: A set of statistical techniques that examines the psychometric properties of measurement instruments

Text mining: The process of extracting and then quantifying and filtering free-text data

Text processing: The process of converting narrative text into structured data for computer processing; *Also called* computer processing of natural language

Textual: A term referring to the narrative nature of much of clinical documentation to date

Theory: A systematic organization of knowledge that predicts or explains the behavior or events

Theory X and Y: A management theory developed by McGregor that describes pessimistic and optimistic assumptions about people and their work potential

Therapeutic privilege: A doctrine that has historically allowed physicians to withhold information from patients in limited circumstances

Therapy threshold: The total number of therapy visits (10) for an episode of care in the Medicare system

Thin client: A computer with processing capability but no persistent storage (disk memory) that relies on data and applications on the host it accesses to be able to process data

Third opinion: Cost containment measure to prevent unnecessary tests, treatments, medical devices, or surgical procedures

Third-party administrator (TPA): An entity that processes healthcare claims and performs related business functions for a health plan

Third-party payer: An insurance company (for example, Blue Cross/Blue Shield) or healthcare program (for example, Medicare) that pays or reimburses healthcare providers (second party) and/or patients (first party) for the delivery of medical services

Third-party payment: Payments for healthcare services made by an insurance company or health agency on behalf of the insured

Threat: 1. The potential for exploitation of a vulnerability 2. Potential danger to a computer, network, or data

Three-dimensional imaging: The construction of pictures generated from computer data in three dimensions

360-degree evaluation: A method of performance evaluation in which the supervisors, peers, and other staff who interact with the employee contribute information

Time and motion studies: Studies in which complex tasks are broken down into their component motions to determine inefficiencies and to develop improvements

Timekeeper: A performance improvement team role responsible for notifying the team during meetings of time remaining on each agenda item in an effort to keep the team moving forward on its performance improvement project

Time ladder: A form used by employees to document time spent on various tasks

Timeliness: 1. The time between the occurrence of an event and the availability of data about the event. Timeliness is related to the use of the data. 2. The completion of a health record within timelines established by legal and accreditation standards and by organizational policy and medical staff bylaws

Time period: A specific span of dates to which data apply

Title: Short name of a diagnosis-related group (DRG), such as DRG 1, Craniotomy Age>17 Except for Trauma

TOB: *See* **type of bill**

Token: 1. A session token is a unique identifier which is generated and sent from a server to a software client to identify an interactive session, and which the client usually stores as an HTTP cookie 2. A security token is usually a physical device that an authorized user of computer services is given to aid in authentication

Toll bypass: A circumvention of the public telephone toll system to avoid the usage fees charged by public carriers

T1: A digital phone line that can carry data at speeds of up to 1.544 megabits per second

Tonometry: The measurement of tension or pressure, especially the indirect estimation of the intraocular pressure, from determination of the resistance of the eyeball to indentation by an applied force

Topography: Code that describes the site of origin of the neoplasm and uses the same three- and four-character categories as in the neoplasm section of the second chapter of ICD-10. Description of a part of the body

Topology: In networking terms, the physical or logical arrangement of a network

Tort: An action brought when one party believes that another party caused harm through wrongful conduct and seeks compensation for that harm

Tort laws: State legislation that applies to civil cases dealing with wrongful conduct or injuries

Total bed count days: The total number of inpatient beds times the total number of days in the period

Total billed charges: All charges for procedures and services rendered to a patient during a hospitalization or encounter

Total discharge days: *See* **total length of stay**

Total inpatient service days: The sum of all inpatient service days for each of the days during a specified period of time

Total length of stay (discharge days): The sum of the days of stay of any group of inpatients discharged during a specific period of time; *See* **discharge days**

Total quality management (TQM): A management philosophy that includes all activities in which the needs of the customer and the organization are satisfied in the most efficient manner by using employee potentials and continuous improvement

TPA: *See* **third-party administrator**

TQM: *See* **total quality management**

Tracer methodology: A process the Joint Commission surveyors use during the on-site survey to analyze an organization's systems, with particular attention to identified priority focus areas, by following individual patients through the organization's healthcare process in the sequence experienced by the patients; an evaluation that follows (traces) the hospital experiences of specific patients to assess the quality of patient care; part of the new Joint Commission survey processes

Traditional fee-for-service (FFS) reimbursement: A reimbursement method involving third-party payers who compensate providers after the healthcare services have been delivered; payment is based on specific services provided to subscribers

Trainee: A person who is learning a task or skill

Trainer: A person who gives instruction on a task or skill

Training: A set of activities and materials that provide the opportunity to acquire job-related skills, knowledge, and abilities

Training and development model: A nine-step plan designed to help the health information manager or human resources department identify the training needs of an employee group

Train-the-trainer: A method of training certain individuals who, in turn, will be responsible for training others on a task or skill

Trait approach: Proposes that leaders possess a collection of traits or qualities that distinguish them from nonleaders

Transactional leadership: Refers to the role of the manager who strives to create an efficient workplace by balancing task accomplishment with interpersonal satisfaction

Transaction and Code Sets rule: Rule designed to standardize transactions performed by healthcare organizations. These standards apply to electronic transactions only; however, paper submissions are similar

Transaction-processing system: A computer-based information system that keeps track of an organization's business transactions through inputs (for example, transaction data such as admissions, discharges, and transfers in a hospital) and outputs (for example, census reports and bills); *Also called* transactional system

Transactions: 1. Units of work performed against a database management system that are treated in a coherent and reliable way independent of other transactions. A database transaction is atomic, consistent, isolated and durable. Examples of healthcare transactions are the entry of a medication order for a patient, the retrieval of a lab result for a patient, and the posting of temperature for a patient 2. The individual events or activities that provide the basic input to the accounting process

Transaction standards: Standards that support the uniform format and sequence of data during transmission from one healthcare entity to another; *See* **transmission standards**

Transcription: The process of deciphering and typing medical dictation

Transcription system: The system can include voice and text functionality. Used by the transcriptionist to listen to and type the various documents dictated by the physicians. The transcription system should be interfaced with the hospital information system so that the patient name, medical record, and date of service are autopopulated within the system

Transcriptionist: A specially trained typist who understands medical terminology and translates physicians' verbal dictation into written reports

Transfer: 1. Moving, without taking out, all or a portion of a body part to another location to take over the function of all or a portion of a body part. The root operation is used to represent those procedures where a body part is moved to another location without disruption of its vascular or nervous supply 2. The movement of a patient from one treatment service or location to another 3. Discharge of a patient from a hospital and readmission to postacute care or another acute care hospital on the same day

Transfer of records: The movement of a record from one medium to another (for example, from paper to microfilm or to an optical imaging system) or to another records custodian

Transfer record: A review of the patient's acute stay along with current status, discharge and transfer orders, and any additional instructions that accompanies the patient when he or she is transferred to another facility; *Also called* a referral form

Transformational leadership: The leadership of a visionary who strives to change an organization

Transfusion reactions: Signs, symptoms, or conditions suffered by a patient as the result of the administration of an incompatible transfusion

Transfusion record: Health record documentation that includes information on the type and amount of blood products a patient received, the source of the blood products, and the patient's reaction to them

Transition: An ongoing plan used in establishing and maintaining the Medicare fee schedule

Transitional facility relative value unit: A blend of charge-based relative value units and resource-based relative expense for services provided in a facility setting

Transitional nonfacility relative value unit: A blend of charge-based relative value units and resource-based relative expense for services provided in a practice setting other than a facility, for example, a physician's office or freestanding clinic

Transmission control protocol/Internet protocol (TCP/IP): The multifaceted protocol suite, or open standard not owned by or proprietary to any company, on which the Internet runs

Transmission standards: Standards that support the uniform format and sequence of data during transmission from one healthcare entity to another; *Also called* **communication standards**; **messaging standards**; *See* **transaction standards**

Transparency: The degree to which individual patients are made aware of how their personal health information is or has been dispersed to secondary medical databases

Transplantation: Putting in or on all or a portion of a living body part taken from another individual or animal to physically take the place and/or function of all or a portion of a similar body part

Trauma center: A hospital that is specially staffed and equipped (usually with an air transport system) to handle trauma patients. They must meet specific criteria for trauma center designation

Trauma registry software: Tracks patients with traumatic injuries from the initial trauma treatment to death

Traumatic injury: A wound or injury included in a trauma registry

Treatment: The manipulation, intervention, or therapy; a broad term used by researchers to generically mean some act, such as a physical conditioning program, a computer training program, a particular laboratory medium, or the timing of prophylactic medications

Treatment guidelines/protocols: *See* **clinical guidelines/protocols**

Treatment, payment, and operations (TPO): Term used in the HIPAA Privacy Rule pertaining to broad activities under normal treatment, payment, and operations activities, important because of the rule's many exceptions to the release and disclosure of personal health information. Collectively, these three actions are functions of a covered entity which are necessary for the covered entity to successfully conduct business

Triage: 1. The sorting of, and allocation of treatment to, patients 2. An early assessment that determines the urgency and priority for care and the appropriate source of care

Trial court: The lowest tier of state court, usually divided into two courts: the court of limited jurisdiction, which hears cases pertaining to a particular subject matter or involving crimes of lesser severity or civil matters of lower dollar amounts; and the court of general jurisdiction, which hears more serious criminal cases or civil cases that involve large amounts of money

TRICARE: The federal healthcare program that provides coverage for the dependents of armed forces personnel and for retirees receiving care outside military treatment facilities in which the federal government pays a percentage of the cost; formerly known as Civilian Health and Medical Program of the Uniformed Services

TRICARE Extra: A healthcare program for standard TRICARE beneficiaries in which they can elect to use a civilian healthcare provider from within the regional contractor's provider network. In this way, TRICARE Extra functions as a preferred provider organization (PPO)

TRICARE for Life (TFL): Secondary coverage for TRICARE beneficiaries who become entitled to Medicare Part A

TRICARE Prime: A TRICARE program that provides the most comprehensive healthcare benefits at the lowest cost of the three TRICARE options, in which military treatment facilities serve as the principal source of healthcare and a primary care manager is assigned to each enrollee

TRICARE Prime Remote: A program that provides active-duty service members in the United States with a specialized version of TRICARE Prime while they are assigned to duty stations in areas not served by the traditional military healthcare system

TRICARE Senior Prime: A managed care demonstration TRICARE program designed to better serve the medical needs of military retirees, dependents, and survivors who are 65 years old and over

TRICARE Standard: A TRICARE program that allows eligible beneficiaries to choose any physician or healthcare provider, which permits the most flexibility but may be the most expensive

Trier of fact: The judge or jury hearing a civil or criminal trial

Trigger: A documented response that alerts a skilled nursing facility resident assessment instrument assessor to the fact that further research is needed to clarify an assessment

Trim point: Numeric value that identifies atypically long lengths of stay (LOS) or high costs (long-stay outliers and cost outliers, respectively); commonly trim points are plus or minus three standard deviations from the mean; *See* **outlier**

Trojan horse: A destructive piece of programming code hidden in another piece of programming code (such as a macro or e-mail message) that looks harmless

TTY: *See* **term type**

Tunneling protocol: A protocol that ensures that data passing over a virtual private network are secure and operates as an outer envelope to an envelope with its enclosure

Turnkey product: A computer application that may be purchased from a vendor and installed without modification or further development by the user organization

Turnkey system: *See* **turnkey product**

Two-tailed hypothesis: A type of alternative hypothesis in which the researcher makes no prediction about the direction of the results

Type of bill (TOB): A form of coding that represents the nature of each form CMS-1450 claim

Type I error: A type of error in which the researcher erroneously rejects the null hypothesis when it is true

Type II error: A type of error in which the researcher erroneously fails to reject the null hypothesis when it is false

Types of requests: The ways in which requests for access, use, and/or disclosure of patient information are made, which may include mail, telephone, physical presence of the requester, fax, e-mail, or other electronic means

UACDS: *See* **Uniform Ambulatory Care Data Set**

UB-04: *See* **Uniform Bill-04**

UB-92 (Uniform Bill-92/CMS-1450): *See* **Uniform Bill-92**

U/C: Usual and customary

UCDS: *See* **Uniform Clinical Data Set**

UCR: *See* **usual, customary, and reasonable**

UDSMR: *See* **Uniform Data Set for Medical Rehabilitation**

UHDDS: *See* **Uniform Hospital Discharge Data Set**

Ultrasound: A diagnostic imaging technique that uses high-frequency, inaudible sound waves that bounce off body tissues. The recorded pattern provides information about the anatomy of an organ

UM: *See* **utilization management; utilization manager**

UMDNS: *See* **Universal Medical Device Nomenclature System**

UML: *See* **unified modeling language**

UMLS: *See* **Unified Medical Language System**

UMLS Knowledge Source Server (UMLSKS): *See* **UMLS Terminology Services**

UMLS Terminology Services (UTS): Replaced the UMLS Knowledge Source Server (UMLSKS) in December 2010. A tool that provides access to the Knowledge Sources and other related resources via the Internet

Unallocated reserves: Monies that have not been assigned a specific use

Unapproved abbreviations policy: A policy that defines the abbreviations that are unacceptable for use in the health record

Unbilled: Specific report that lists patient encounters that have ended but for whom a final bill has not been prepared

Unbilled account: An account that has not been billed and is not included in accounts receivable

Unbundling: The practice of using multiple codes to bill for the various individual steps in a single procedure rather than using a single code that includes all of the steps of the comprehensive procedure

Uncontrollable costs: Costs over which department managers have little or no influence

Undercoding: A form of incomplete documentation that results when diagnoses or procedures that should be coded are not assigned

Understandable, reproducible, and useful (URU) principle: The guiding principle for modeling concepts in SNOMED CT, which states that all concepts must be understandable, reproducible, and useful

Unfavorable variance: The negative difference between the budgeted amount and the actual amount of a line item, where actual revenue is less than budget or where actual expenses exceed budget

Unfreezing: The first stage of Lewin's change process in which people are presented with disconcerting information to motivate them to change

Unified Medical Language System (UMLS): A program initiated by the National Library of Medicine to build an intelligent, automated system that can understand biomedical concepts, words, and expressions and their interrelationships; includes concepts and terms from many different source vocabularies

Unified Medical Language System (UMLS) Metathesaurus: A list containing information on biomedical concepts and terms from more than 100 healthcare vocabularies and classifications, administrative health data, bibliographic and full-text databases, and expert systems

Unified Medical Language System (UMLS) Semantic Network: A categorization of all concepts UMDNS in the UMLS Metathesaurus

Unified Medical Language System (UMLS) SPECIALIST Lexicon: An English-language lexicon containing biomedical terms

Unified messaging: The ability for an individual to receive and/or retrieve various forms of messaging at a single access point, including voice, e-mail, fax, and text messages

Unified modeling language (UML): A common data-modeling notation used in conjunction with object-oriented database design

Uniform Ambulatory Care Data Set (UACDS): A data set developed by the National Committee on Vital and Health Statistics consisting of a minimum set of patient- or client-specific data elements to be collected in ambulatory care settings

Uniform Bill-04 (UB-04): The single standardized Medicare form for standardized uniform billing, implemented in 2007 for hospital inpatients and outpatients;

this form will also be used by the major third-party payers and most hospitals

Uniform Bill-92 (UB-92): Replaced by the UB-04 in 2007; it was a Medicare form for standardized uniform billing

Uniform Code on Dental Procedures and Nomenclatures: *See* **Current Dental Terminology**

Uniformed Services Employment and Reemployment Rights Act (1994): Federal legislation that prohibits discrimination against individuals because of their service in the uniformed services

Uniform Hospital Discharge Data Set (UHDDS): A core set of data elements adopted by the US Department of Health, Education, and Welfare in 1974 that are collected by hospitals on all discharges and all discharge abstract systems

Uniform Resource Locator (URL): A unique website address that will take the web browser directly to the document located on a web page

UNII Codes: *See* **Established Name for Active Ingredients and FDA Unique Ingredient Identifier Codes**

Union: A collective bargaining unit that represents groups of employees and is authorized to negotiate with employers on the employees' behalf in matters related to compensation, health, and safety; *Also called* **labor organization**

Unique identification number: A combination of numbers or alphanumeric characters assigned to a particular patient

Unique identifier: A type of information that refers to only one individual or organization

Unique personal identifier: A unique number assigned by a healthcare provider to a patient that distinguishes the patient and his or her medical record from all others in the institution, assists in the retrieval of the record, and facilitates the posting of payment

Unique physician identification number (UPIN): A unique numerical identifier created by the Centers for Medicare and Medicaid Services for use by physicians who bill for services provided to Medicare patients. Discontinued in 2007 and replaced with the National Provider Identifier (NPI)

Unique user identifier: A unique identifier assigned to all authorized users of the health record and used to track users and log-in procedures

United Nations International Standards Organization (ISO): An international standards organization that coordinates all international standards development

Unit filing system: A health record filing system in which all inpatient and outpatient visits and procedures are arranged together under a permanent unit number

Unit labor cost: Cost determined by dividing the total annual compensation by total annual productivity

Unit numbering system: A health record identification system in which the patient receives a unique medical record number at the time of the first encounter that is used for all subsequent encounters

Unit testing: The testing step in EHR implementation that ensures that each data element is captured, recorded, and processed appropriately within a given application

Unit work division: A method of work organization where each task is performed by one person at the same time that another person is doing a task, but one does not have to wait for the other

Unity of command: A human resources principle that assumes that each employee reports to only one specific management position

Univariate: A term referring to the involvement of one variable

Universal chart order: A system in which the health record is maintained in the same format while the patient is in the facility and after discharge

Universal Medical Device Nomenclature System (UMDNS): A standard international nomenclature and computer coding system for medical devices, developed by ECRI

Universal patient identifier: A personal identifier applied to a patient, such as a number or code, that is used permanently for many and varied purposes

Universal personal identifier: A concept whereby a unique numerical identifier is assigned to individual recipients of healthcare services in the United States

Universal precautions: The application of a set of procedures specifically designed to minimize or eliminate the passage of infectious disease agents from one individual to another during the provision of healthcare services

Universal protocol: A written checklist developed by the Joint Commission to prevent errors that can occur when physicians perform the wrong procedure, for example

UNIX: An operating system developed by AT&T's Bell Laboratories in 1969, and one of the best systems for mission-critical applications

Unlisted procedure codes: Codes available in each section of CPT to describe procedures that have no specific procedure code assigned because the procedure is new or unusual

Unrestricted question: A type of question that allows free-form responses; *Also called* **open-ended question**

Unsecured personal health information (PHI): Personal health information that has not been rendered unusable, unreadable, or indecipherable to unauthorized persons

Unstructured brainstorming method: A group problem-solving technique wherein the team leader solicits spontaneous ideas for the topic under discussion from members of the team in a free-flowing and nonjudgmental manner

Unstructured data: Nonbinary, human-readable data

Unstructured decision: A decision that is made without following a prescribed method, formula, or pattern

Unstructured question: A type of question that allows free-form responses; *See* **open-ended question**

Unsupervised learning: Any learning technique that has as its purpose to group or cluster items, objects, or individuals

Upcoding: The practice of assigning diagnostic or procedural codes that represent higher payment rates than the codes that actually reflect the services provided to patients; *See* **overcoding**

Update: The annual adjustment to the Medicare fee schedule conversion factor

UPIN: *See* **unique physician identification number**

UPP: Urethral pressure profile

UR: *See* **utilization review**

Urban area: A metropolitan statistical area as defined by the Office of Management and Budget; *See* **core-based statistical area (CBSA)**

Urgent admission: An admission in which the patient requires immediate attention for care and treatment of a physical or psychiatric problem. Generally, the patient is admitted to the first available, suitable accommodation

URL: *See* **Uniform Resource Locator**

URU principle: *See* **Understandable, reproducible, and useful (URU) principle**

Use case: A technique that develops scenarios based on how users will use information to assist in developing information systems that support the information requirements

Use case diagram: A systems analysis technique used to document a software project from a user's perspective

Use, disclosures, and requests: Three types of situations in which personal health information is handled: use, which is internal to a covered entity or its business associate; disclosure, which is the dissemination of PHI from a covered entity or its business associate; and requests for PHI made by a covered entity or its business associate

User-based access: A security mechanism used to grant users of a system access based on identity

User groups: Groups composed of users of a particular computer system

Uses and disclosures: Referring to the use and disclosure of a patient's personal health information

US Public Health Service: An agency of the US Department of Health and Human Services that promotes the protection and advancement of physical and mental health

Usual, customary, and reasonable (UCR): Type of retrospective fee-for-service payment method in which the third-party payer pays for fees that are usual, customary, and reasonable, wherein "usual" is usual for the individual provider's practice; "customary" means customary for the community; and "reasonable" is reasonable for the situation

Usual, customary, and reasonable (UCR) charges: Method of evaluating providers' fees in which the third-party payer pays for fees that are "usual" in that provider's practice; "customary" in the community; and "reasonable" for the situation

Usual fee: The amount a physician normally charges the majority of the patients seen for that service

Utility program: A software program that supports, enhances, or expands existing programs in a computer system, such as virus checking, data recovery, backup, and data compression

Utilization: Patterns of usage for a single medical service or type of service

Utilization management (UM): 1. A collection of systems and processes to ensure that facilities and resources, both human and nonhuman, are used maximally and are consistent with patient care needs 2. A program that evaluates the healthcare facility's efficiency in providing necessary care to patients in the most effective manner

Utilization management organization: An organization that reviews the appropriateness of the care setting and resources used to treat a patient

Utilization manager (UM): Person that evaluates patient care, ensuring neither underutilization nor overutilization of resources

Utilization review (UR): The process of determining whether the medical care provided to a specific patient is necessary according to preestablished objective screening criteria at time frames specified in the organization's utilization management plan

Utilization Review Act: The federal legislation that requires hospitals to conduct continued-stay reviews for Medicare and Medicaid patients

UTS: *See* **UMLS Terminology Services**

Validity: 1. The extent to which data correspond to the actual state of affairs or that an instrument measures what it purports to measure 2. A term referring to a test's ability to accurately and consistently measure what it purports to measure

Valuation: The estimated market value of a project, an object, a merger, and so on

Value-based leadership: An approach that emphasizes values, ethics, and stewardship as central to effective leadership

Value-based purchasing (VBP): CMS incentive plan that links payments more directly to the quality of care provided and rewards providers for delivering high-quality and efficient clinical care. It incorporates clinical process-of-care measures as well as measures from the Hospital Consumer Assessment of Healthcare Providers and Systems (HCAHPS) survey on how patients view their care experiences

Value set: A collection of concepts drawn from one or more vocabulary code systems and grouped together for a specific purpose

Values statement: A short description that communicates an organization's social and cultural belief system

Variability: The dispersion of a set of measures around the population mean

Variable: A characteristic or property that may take on different values

Variable costs: Resources expended that vary with the activity of the organization, for example, medication expenses vary with patient volume

Variance: A disagreement between two parts; the square of the standard deviation; a measure of variability that gives the average of the squared deviations from the mean; in financial management, the difference between the budgeted amount and the actual amount of a line item; in project management, the difference between the original project plan and current estimates

Variance analysis: An assessment of a department's financial transactions to identify differences between the budget amount and the actual amount of a line item

Vascular family: A group of blood vessels that is fed by a branch, or primary division, of a major blood vessel

Vascular order: The furthest point to which the catheter is placed into the branches of a vessel originating off the aorta, vena cava, or vessel punctured if the aorta is not entered, and is referred to the level of selectivity

VBAC: The acronym for vaginal birth after a previous cesarean delivery

VBP: *See* **value-based purchasing**

V codes: A set of ICD-9-CM codes used to classify occasions when circumstances other than disease or injury are recorded as the reason for the patient's encounter with healthcare providers

Vector graphic data: Digital data that have been captured as points and are connected by lines (a series of point coordinates) or areas (shapes bounded by lines); *Also called* **signal tracing data**

Vendors: Companies that provide products and/or services to healthcare organizations. Depending upon access to protected health information (PHI), the vendor may or may not be categorized as a business associate

Vendor system: A computer system developed by a commercial company not affiliated with the healthcare organization

Verification: The act of proving or disproving the subject matter or documents in question or comparing an activity, a process, or a product with the corresponding requirements or specifications

Verification service: An outside service that provides a primary source check on information that a physician makes available on an application to the medical staff

Version control: The process whereby a healthcare facility ensures that only the most current version of a patient's health record is available for viewing, updating, and so forth

Vertical dyad linkage: *See* **leader–member exchange**

Vertically integrated plan: *See* **integrated provider organization**

Vertically integrated system: *See* **integrated provider organization**

Vertical structure: The levels and relationships among positions in an organizational hierarchy

Veterans Health Administration: The component of the US Department of Veterans Affairs that implements the medical assistance program of the VA

Videoconferencing: A communications service that allows a group of people to exchange information over a network by using a combination of video and computer technology

Virtual HIM: Health information management function that takes place outside of a traditional office setting

Virtual private network (VPN): An encrypted tunnel through the Internet that enables secure transmission of data

Virtual reality (VR): An artificial form of reality experienced through sensory stimuli and in which the participant's actions partly affect what happens

Virus: A computer program, typically hidden, that attaches itself to other programs and has the ability to replicate and cause various forms of harm to the data

Vision: A picture of the desired future that sets a direction and rationale for change

Vision statement: A short description of an organization's ideal future state

Visit: A single encounter with a healthcare professional that includes all of the services supplied during the encounter

Vital statistics: Data related to births, deaths, marriages, and fetal deaths

Vitrectomy: An ocular surgical procedure involving removal of the soft jelly-like material (vitreous humor) that fills the area behind the lens of the eye (vitreous chamber) and replacement with a clear solution. This is necessary when blood and scar tissue accumulate in the vitreous humor

VLBW: Very low birth weight

Vocabulary mapping process: A process that connects one clinical vocabulary to another

Vocabulary standards: A list or collection of clinical words or phrases with their meanings; also, the set of words used by an individual or group within a particular subject field; *See* **controlled vocabulary**

Vocational rehabilitation: The evaluation and training aimed at assisting a person to enter or reenter the labor force

Voiceover IP (VoIP): *See* **Internet protocol technology**

Voice recognition technology: A method of encoding speech signals that do not require speaker pauses (but uses pauses when they are present) and of interpreting at least some of the signals' content as words or the intent of the speaker; *See* **continuous speech technology**

VoIP: *See* **Internet protocol technology**

Voir dire: The process of jury selection

Volume logs: Forms used (sometimes in conjunction with time ladders) to obtain information about the volume of work units received and processed in a day

Voluntary Disclosure Program: A program unveiled in 1998 by OIG that encourages healthcare providers to voluntarily report fraudulent conduct affecting Medicare, Medicaid, and other federal healthcare programs

Voluntary review: An examination of an organization's structures and processes conducted at the request of a healthcare facility seeking accreditation from a reviewing agency

VPN: *See* **virtual private network**

V/Q: Ventilation-perfusion

Vulnerability: An inherent weakness or absence of a safeguard that could be exploited by a threat

W

Wage index: Ratio that represents the relationship between the average wages in a healthcare setting's geographic area and the national average for that healthcare setting. Wage indexes are adjusted annually and published in the *Federal Register*

Waiting period: Time between the effective date of a healthcare insurance policy and the date the healthcare insurance plan will assume liability for expenses related to certain health services, such as those related to pre-existing conditions

Waiver: *See* **advance beneficiary notice**

Waiver of privilege: An exception to physician–patient privilege that occurs when a party claims damages for a mental or physical injury; the party thereby waives his or her right to confidentiality to the extent that it is necessary to determine whether the mental or physical injury is due to another cause

WAN: *See* **wide-area network**

Web appliance: A computer without secondary storage capability that is designed to connect to a network

Web-based systems and applications: Systems and applications that use Internet technology

Web-based training: Instruction via the Internet that enables individuals to learn in a structure that is self-paced and self-directed while interacting and collaborating with other students and the instructor via a conferencing system

Web browser-based (or web native) architectures: *See* **web browser-based systems**

Web browser-based systems: Systems and applications written in one or more web programming languages; *Also called* **web browser-based (or web native) architectures**

Web content management systems: Systems in which information placed on a website can be labeled and tracked so that it can be easily located, modified, and reused

Web-enabled technology: An application that was originally written for a client or server or mainframe environment that is rewritten to be accessed through a web browser

Webmasters: Individuals who support web applications and the healthcare organization's intranet and Internet operations

Web portal: A website entryway through which to access, find, and deliver information

Web portal technology: A website entryway serving as a starting point to access, find, and deliver information and including a broad array of resources and services, such as e-mail, forums, and search engines

Web services: An open, standardized way of integrating disparate, web browser-based and other applications

Web services architecture (WSA): An architecture that utilizes web-based tools to permit communication among different software applications

WEDI: *See* **Workgroup on Electronic Data Interchange**

Weight: The numerical assignment that is part of the formula by which a specific dollar amount, or reimbursement, is calculated for each diagnosis-related group or each ambulatory payment classification

Well newborn: A newborn born at term, under sterile conditions, with no diseases, conditions, disorders, syndromes, injuries, malformations, or defects diagnosed, and no operations other than routine circumcisions performed

Western blot test: A blood test used to diagnose infection with human immunodeficiency virus (HIV)

WHO: *See* **World Health Organization**

Whole number: Any of the set of nonnegative integers. It cannot be a fraction, decimal, percentage, or negative number

WICC: *See* **Wonca International Classification Committee**

Wide-area network (WAN): A computer network that connects devices across a large geographical area

Wired equivalent privacy (WEP): A form of encryption used to authenticate the sender and receiver of messages over networks, particularly when the Internet is involved in the data transmission; should provide authentication (both sender and recipient are known to each other), data security (safe from interception), and data nonrepudiation (data that were sent have arrived unchanged)

Wireless local-area network (WLAN): A wireless local-area network that uses radio waves as the carrier

Wireless on wheels (WOWs): Notebook computers mounted on carts that can be moved through the facility by users

Wireless technology: A type of technology that uses wireless networks and wireless devices to access and transmit data in real time

Wireless wide-area network (WWAN): Network that uses mobile telecommunication cellular network technologies to connect computers across a large area

Withhold: Portion of providers' capitated payments that managed care organizations deduct and hold in order to create an incentive for efficient or reduced utilization of healthcare services; *Also called* **physician contingency reserve**

Withhold pool: Aggregate amount withheld from all providers' capitation payments as an amount to cover expenditures in excess of targets

WLAN: *See* **wireless local-area network**

Wonca: *See* **World Organization of Family Doctors**

Wonca International Classification Committee (WICC): The current name of the Wonca Classification Committee, the group that designed the International Classification of Primary Care

WORK: *See* **physician work**

Work: The effort, usually described in hours, needed to complete a task

Work and data flow analyst: The work and data flow analyst must be able to study the flow of data into the system and its associated processes and look for ways to improve it, using data flow diagrams and other tools to document the various flows of data within the facility

Work breakdown structure: A hierarchical structure that decomposes project activities into levels of detail

Work distribution analysis: An analysis used to determine whether a department's current work assignments and job content are appropriate

Work distribution chart: A matrix that depicts the work being done in a particular workgroup in terms of specific tasks and activities, time spent on tasks, and the employees performing the tasks

Work division: The way in which tasks are handled within an organization

Workflow: Any work process that must be handled by more than one person

Workflow analysis: A technique used to study the flow of operations for automation; *See* **operations analysis**

Workflow technology: Technology that automatically routes electronic documents into electronic in-baskets of its department staff for disposition decisions

Workforce: Under the HIPAA Privacy Rule, employees, volunteers, trainees, and other persons whether paid or not who work for and are under the direct control of the covered entity

Workforce members: Employees, volunteers, trainees, and other persons who work under the direct control of a HIPAA-covered entity, regardless of whether they are paid by the covered entity

Workforce trends: Referring to changes that will likely take place in the workforce in the future

Workgroup on Electronic Data Interchange (WEDI): A subgroup of Accreditation Standards Committee X12 that has been involved in developing electronic data interchange standards for billing transactions

Work imaging study: A technique used to analyze the time required of full-time equivalent employees (FTEs) compared with established productivity standards

Work measurement: The process of studying the amount of work accomplished and how long it takes to accomplish work in order to define and monitor productivity

Work products: Documents produced during the completion of a task that may be a component of, or contribute to, a project deliverable

Work sampling: A work measurement technique that uses random sample measurements to characterize the performance of the whole

Work schedules: The process by which facility managers ensure that each department has adequate personnel to properly complete all assigned tasks

Workaround: A temporary alternate process created as a substitute for an undesirable process to achieve a desired outcome until a more permanent solution is found

Workers' Adjustment and Retraining Notification (WARN) Act: Federal legislation that requires employers to give employees a 60-day notice in advance of covered plant closings and covered mass layoffs

Worker Immaturity–Maturity: The model developed by Argyris to describe how leadership should change with an employee's maturity

Workers' compensation: The medical and income insurance coverage for certain employees in unusually hazardous jobs

Working conditions: The environment in which work is performed (surroundings) and the physical dangers or risks involved in performing the job (hazards)

Workstation: A computer designed to accept data from multiple sources in order to assist in managing information for daily activities and to provide a convenient means of entering data as desired by the user at the point of care

World Health Organization (WHO): The United Nations specialized agency created to ensure the attainment by all peoples of the highest possible levels of health; responsible for a number of international classifications, including the International Statistical Classification of Diseases & Related Health Problems (ICD-10) and the International Classification of Functioning, Disability & Health (ICF)

World Organization of Family Doctors (Wonca): The organization instrumental in the development of the International Classification of Primary Care; formerly called the World Organization of National Colleges, Academics, and Academic Associations of General Practitioners/Family Physicians (Wonca)

World Wide Web (www): A global network of networks offering services to users with web browsers

Worm: A special type of computer virus, usually transferred from computer to computer via e-mail, that can replicate itself and use memory but cannot attach itself to other programs

WORM technology: Write once, read many. The use of this technology prevents the user from altering what is stored, but the data can be viewed as many times as necessary

Wound repair: Refers to three types of repair: *simple*, which refers to the repair of superficial wounds, involving primarily epidermis or dermis or subcutaneous tissues without significant involvement of deeper structures; *intermediate,* which involves the repair of wounds that require layered closure of one or more of the deeper layers of subcutaneous tissues and superficial (non-muscle) fascia, in addition to the skin (epidermal and dermal) closure; and *complex*, which designates the repair of wounds requiring more than layered closures, namely, scar revision, debridement, extensive undermining, stents, or retention sutures

Write-off: The action taken to eliminate the balance of a bill after the bill has been submitted and partial payment has been made or payment has been denied and all avenues of collecting the payment have been exhausted

WSA: *See* **web services architecture**

X-axis: The horizontal axis on a graph where the independent variables are noted

XML: *See* **extensible markup language**

X12: An ANSI-accredited group that defines EDI standards for many American industries, including healthcare insurance. Most of the electronic transaction standards mandated or proposed under HIPAA are X12 standards

X12N: A subcommittee of X12 that defines EDI standards for the insurance industry, including healthcare insurance

***Y*-axis:** The vertical axis on a graph that displays frequency

Years of schooling: The highest grade of schooling completed by the enrollee or patient

Zero balance: The result of writing off the balance of an account, which closes off the account and ends the days in accounts receivable

Zero-based budgets: Types of budgets in which each budget cycle poses the opportunity to continue or discontinue services based on available resources so that every department or activity must be justified and prioritized annually to effectively allocate resources

Zip: A computer utility that combines two or more files into one and reduces the size of the file

Zone program integrity contractor (ZPIC): A CMS program that replaces the Medicare Program Safeguard Contractors (PSCs). ZPICs are responsible for detection and prevention of fraud, waste, and abuse across all Medicare claim types by performing medical reviews, data analysis, and auditing

ZPIC: *See* **Zone program integrity contractor**